THE THREE RULES TO LOSE WEIGHT AND KEEP IT OFF FOREVER

LIVE BETTER AND EAT AS MUCH AS YOU WANT WITHOUT COUNTING CARBS

HAROLD OSTER, MD

To Angie and Troy, the best people I know. And to Ryan Holiday, whose books changed my life.

CONTENTS

Preface to the Second Edition

If at first...

In 2020, I published the first edition of *The Three Rules to Lose Weight and Keep It Off Forever*. The plan works, and I'm happy with the results. Patients, friends, and strangers have told me how much weight they have lost and how they're happier and healthier. As I expected, some have told me that the diet is too difficult, that they can't give up certain foods, and that they don't want to put in the effort it takes to follow The Rules. To them, I usually say, "Do it anyway."

In this edition, I add the immortal words of Stephen Covey in *The Seven Habits of Highly Effective People,* "Begin with the end in mind." Decide what your goals are and aim for them. If your goal is to lose all your extra weight and keep it off, follow The Three Rules as closely as possible. If not, then take what works for you from the book and disregard the rest. Make a plan and establish a goal.

My mind works best with all or none—follow The Rules or don't. But I've learned since writing *The Three Rules to Lose Weight and Keep It Off Forever* that some people benefit even if their minds work differently. My son has decided (for now) to follow The Rules most of the time, taking breaks to eat certain prohibited foods. If he gains a few pounds, he'll restart the plan. I've tried this approach many times and failed, but perhaps I was arrogant, thinking that no one could do it and succeed. Time will tell how successful my son is. I believe, though, that most people act as if they are addicted to what I call bad carbs. In the last fifty years, our lives have become so convenient, and bad carbs are so easily obtained that acting as if bad carbs are an addiction and approaching it with total abstinence is the best approach for most of us. The Three Rules will help anyone lose weight and keep it off—those who accept abstinence as the answer and those who want a more nuanced approach. But I prefer abstinence.

Since I wrote the first edition, more studies have confirmed the harms of bad carbohydrates and the benefits of avoiding them. New weight loss drugs have become available, some with significant promise. Products with "keto" on their labels have appeared in grocery stores, and restaurants are putting "keto-friendly" on their menus. More labels say "zero sugar" than ever before. I will help you determine which foods are worth eating and which will ruin your plans.

The Three Rules haven't changed, but as with everything, the world has changed around it. In some ways, for those with discipline, losing weight on my plan is more manageable than before—there are more healthy options. But with these choices, we must be careful.

I recently retired from medicine. Since graduating from medical school so many years ago, I have seen Americans' weight steadily increase. I now believe that obesity is the paramount health problem in the United States. *The Three Rules to Lose Weight and Keep It Off*

Forever has helped me and my patients take control of their weight. I hope it helps you.

Harold Oster, 2024

Preface to the First Edition: How I Discovered the Rules

It took me three decades, but I figured it out.

I excel at losing weight. I am better at gaining it. The Three Rules is not a scheme to lose weight quickly; it will help you lose weight and keep it off forever. This book is for people like me, people willing to work hard at something important. Losing weight is hard, and keeping it off is hard. But you can do it. The Three Rules to Lose Weight and Keep It Off Forever will help you.

My approach to self-improvement has changed over my life. I am trying to live the values of the Stoics who lived around two thousand years ago. If you know little about Stoicism, it differs from what you imagined. It doesn't teach us to be unemotional and hard-hearted; it teaches us how to live our best lives. My first real exposure to Stoicism was when I read *The Obstacle Is the Way* by Ryan Holiday. Holiday teaches that we become better by confronting and overcoming obstacles. The Three Rules to Lose Weight and Keep It Off *Forever* embraces the same philosophy. Anyone can overcome the obstacle of weight control by following The Rules in this book. It is hard; it's an obstacle, but you can surmount it. You will be better for it.

I am working to become healthier and to stay healthy for as long as possible. The most important step has been to lose weight and keep it off. In medical school, we didn't learn much about obesity. It was nowhere near as common as now, though we saw obese patients. Obesity was not a very important topic. We learned about obesity-related illnesses, such as diabetes and heart failure, but the professors didn't stress the causes and treatments of obesity. They taught us that if you overeat, you will gain weight. If you cut back and exercise, you will lose weight. That's true, as far as it goes. But why do so many people struggle? Why is obesity becoming more common if everyone knows why we gain weight, and everyone knows how to lose it?

As a kid, I thought doctors were doctors, pilots were pilots, and plumbers were plumbers. They were not regular people. Now I know that everyone in every profession has their own life, and even doctors can be overweight or thin, healthy or sick. My struggle was always my weight and control over my eating. I gained and lost weight many times over many years, and when I became a physician, I saw my patients struggle similarly. Over time, I developed various strategies for my patients and myself, and I have settled on the Three Rules as the best approach for most people. What I didn't learn in medical school, I learned in my life and in the office with my patients.

Losing weight has countless benefits. You will feel better, have more opportunities to enjoy life, and be healthier. Yes, it is hard to lose weight. If it were easy, there wouldn't be an obesity problem, and there would be no demand for books like this. Anyone who tells you otherwise is wrong or lying. As the saying goes, nothing worth doing is easy.

Some health problems require medications or surgery, just as some projects at home require an expert. Medical intervention has a role in weight management, but only if you have tried everything first. You can lose weight and keep it off on your own if you work hard enough. I don't believe the clichés that anyone can do absolutely anything they set out to do if they work hard. I could never play NBA basketball or become a chess grandmaster. But I believe anyone can lose weight. It is hard. Do it anyway.

I Know How to Lose Weight

When I was young, I was healthy and somewhat athletic, and I ate well. I was never obese but was consistently up a few pounds, and I was never as lean as my brother. A few times in high school, I tried to lose weight and was somewhat successful. Too many lunches at Burger King with my best friend always led to a rapid return to my previous weight. In my first year of medical school at the University of Miami, I stress-ate and found myself 20 pounds overweight on a five-foot, five-inch frame. I started a diet.

This first real diet was low-calorie. Low-calorie diets are typically low-fat since fat has more calories per gram than anything else. I mostly ate salads at Burger King and small meals at home. A snack was a piece of bread, sometimes toasted. I didn't enjoy it and was hungry most of the time. But it worked—I lost weight. The following year, I was heavy again, mainly from the exquisite chicken sandwich and fries at Wendy's, located conveniently near the University of Miami library. A few months later, I dieted again with calorie-cutting, was again hungry most of the time, and lost another

20 pounds. I kept track of my weight in a little green notebook, in which I also recorded interesting medical facts, complex formulas, and phone numbers. Over the next several years, I gained weight and then dieted, always with the same hunger. But it always worked because I was disciplined. It was stressful, and I was always hungry, but it worked.

In 1996, I was around 25 pounds overweight and about to start a tough rotation of my fellowship training in Infectious Diseases at Mount Sinai Hospital in Miami Beach. I wanted to lose weight, but I knew I'd have difficulty being hungry during stressful, long days. Then, I learned of *Dr. Atkins' New Diet Revolution*. Robert Atkins did not invent the low-carbohydrate diet, but he brought it to public attention. He believed cutting out virtually all carbohydrates leads to weight loss without hunger. He was right. The diet works, and there are few health risks, at least in the short term.

Over the next six weeks, I got to the hospital cafeteria very early, had breakfast, and planned my long day of seeing patients. Usually, I ate an omelet and sausage or ham. After seeing patients all morning, I had lunch: cheeseburgers without the bun, chicken salad, tuna salad, eggs, cheese, and anything low in carbohydrates and high in protein and fat. I worked through the afternoon and evening, regularly arriving home after 8:00 p.m. Dinner was steak, fried Spam (my favorite), or chicken, and often more eggs and cheese. I lost 25 pounds in six weeks, and I was never hungry.

After the rotation, I felt I could just eat sensibly, in moderation. It worked for a while, but soon, I resumed my old habits—snacks, bread, and fast food. In less than six months, I was again 20 pounds overweight. I have since misplaced my green notebook with the details, but I gained and lost weight multiple times over the next six or eight years. (I treasured that notebook.) Mostly, I did the Atkins Diet because giving up carbohydrates (from now on, I will usually say carbs) while eating more protein and fat was easier for me than hunger. But every time, after I completed the diet, thinking I could eat my usual food in moderation, I gained the weight back. I didn't realize the obvious—I could not eat sensibly. I couldn't eat junk food and carbs in moderation.

What ended my use of the Atkins Diet is not an issue for most people. Worried about the health effects, I had my cholesterol checked. Healthy total cholesterol is under 200. Mine was over 475, and my LDL, the so-called bad cholesterol, was about 400, more than triple the recommended level. I had the tests repeated and spoke to an expert on the effects of the Atkins Diet. He said this rise in cholesterol was uncommon, and he asked me to stay on the diet and have my blood sent to him to determine if I was a hyper-absorber of cholesterol. I told him to forget it, not wanting another day of a cholesterol level that high. Since then, I have confirmed in reading and with my patients that most people don't have a significant rise in cholesterol on the diet.

After a few more times gaining and losing weight (back exclusively to calorie-cutting and hunger), I was frustrated. At about that time, *The South Beach Diet*, by Arthur Agatston, MD (from the same hospital where I first tried the Atkins Diet), became popular. This diet cuts most carbohydrates but allows for many fruits and vegetables, and later in the diet, some bread and other foods with moderate carbohydrate content. Unlike the Atkins Diet, it encourages lean protein and healthy fats. I did okay with this diet, and my cholesterol didn't rise, but I struggled when the diet called for moderation. It allows for certain foods in prescribed amounts, and I couldn't always stop eating when I reached the permitted limits. I lost weight, though not as quickly as with the Atkins Diet, and I always gained it back.

In 2004, my wife, son, and I moved to Minnesota to be closer to family. I had already lost twenty pounds or more at least fifteen times. Over the next five to ten years, I gained and lost weight several more times and began to notice the same pattern in some of my patients. Most people become frustrated with the food deprivations and hunger associated with weight loss, and if they do lose weight, rapid regaining typically follows.

Allina Health, the company I worked for, started a program to improve employees' fitness, including that of physicians. Since I already knew I was overweight, I figured the program wouldn't help me. In many studies, programs such as ours make little difference in the participants' overall health. Our program included a fat percentage test. It's not perfectly accurate, but it told me what I already knew—I was fat. Seeing the number in print put to rest any of the stories we tell ourselves—we have more muscle than fat, we're big-boned, and so on. I decided enough was enough. My bad carbohydrate and junk food habit was like any other, and to succeed, I had to give it up entirely.

Since that day, I have vowed to give up junk food. But what does that mean? I realized I needed a way of eating that was simple and that I could do forever. I wanted concrete guidelines of what to eat and what to eliminate. I realized carbohydrates were the problem because starving myself is too difficult, and studies show calorie-cutting leads to muscle loss. But the Atkins Diet is too restrictive, and the South Beach Diet is complicated, eliminating some carbs but allowing for others in moderation, which is too difficult. There are many other diet programs, but they have similar shortcomings. My troubles taught me that simple, concrete rules are necessary. I devised a plan that covered all my requirements, and my weight has been normal since.

I Know Why My Patients Did Not Succeed

As I struggled with my weight issues, the nation as a whole was getting heavier. Over the years, the average body mass index, a measure of a person's weight against their height, with 30.0 defining obesity and 25.0 defining overweight, has increased dramatically. My panel of patients reflected the national trends. I talked to obese patients about the problem nearly every visit, but as a rule, they didn't lose weight. I was surprised, but most just did not put forth the required effort; they didn't realize how much work it takes. There were a few who worked hard and were able to lose weight, but they usually gained it back just as quickly as I had.

My recommendations to my patients mirrored what I was doing for my own weight problem. I started out recommending cutting calories, but no one liked going hungry, and no one liked giving up the high-calorie foods they enjoyed. Unfortunately, those who managed to lose weight by eating less usually lost significant muscle mass. As I learned the value of carbohydrate control, I recommended it more and more, usually with the Atkins Diet. When patients diligently stuck to the Atkins Diet, they lost weight, but they typically quit before reaching their goal because the diet was too restrictive. Then, they quickly regained what they'd lost. I still believe in the value of the Atkins Diet, but only for the severely obese; it allows them to lose some weight rapidly and feel a sense of accomplishment.

I then moved to the South Beach Diet and other similar diet plans, which some call modified Atkins Diets. I tried to convince my patients to lose weight by giving them diet summaries and recommending a few books. Some patients took my advice seriously and even bought the books. But they usually felt the plans were too complicated with too many things to remember. They had to learn lists and measure serving sizes and thought they couldn't stick to the diets outside their home.

I kept at it, knowing that carbohydrates were the key. (Later in this book, I will detail why carbohydrate-based plans work.) But people need a simple, inexpensive plan they can follow without weighing and measuring food, a program allowing them to eat at restaurants and with their friends and family. Over several years, I frequently changed my instructions, telling patients to avoid diets with multiple stages, eliminate any foods that needed to be measured, and stop buying expensive packaged diet foods. I gave patients lists of prohibited foods and recommended more books to read. Slowly, more and more people lost weight. But still, most didn't, and the majority who lost weight regained it. The diets were still too complicated and seemed too restrictive. Regardless of the method, losing weight is difficult.

The diet I was following worked. It eliminated nearly everything my patients and I disliked about calorie-cutting and carbohydrate-based diets, everything that leads to failure, frustration, and relapse. I converted my diet into simple rules that, when followed, lead to success. I whittled my rules down to three and changed the wording about twenty times. I gave patients summaries of the diet and told them how to do it. They could still enjoy eating, eat with friends, eat at restaurants, and eat inexpensively. I taught everyone who would listen about my plan, The Three Rules to Lose Weight and Keep It Off Forever.

This plan was still an effort, and most patients didn't even start it. I understood why, and I didn't blame them. It's easier to eat whatever we want, when we want. It's easier to make small efforts, but small efforts and half-measures don't work. You must have excellent reasons to work hard at something, but if you put in the effort, The Three Rules plan works. Once in a while, a patient took me up on it, applying The Three Rules to their lives. These people succeeded.

As I was writing the first edition, I saw a patient with diabetes. When I had seen him a few months before, his sugars were okay but not great, and he was taking two medications. I had told him about The Three Rules at earlier visits and reviewed it again. He took it to heart and started the plan. This time, he came in having lost twenty pounds—his weight was nearly normal, and he looked fit. His labs showed completely normal sugars. Most patients didn't put in the effort, but when they did, The Rules worked. The complete resolution of his diabetes was not a surprise. Studies show that about 90% of people with diabetes who lose most or all their excess weight go into remission, meaning there is no sign of diabetes on lab tests. Most go off medication completely, and I stopped one of this patient's medications at that visit.

I have taught my son that you should almost never say never or always. So, I will say only this: those who follow the Three Rules to Lose Weight and Keep It Off Forever will almost always be successful. Some people may follow The Three Rules closely and not lose weight, but I have yet to see it. It almost never fails.

What to Expect in This Book

Over thirty years of struggling with my weight (and nearly as long seeing patients struggle) led to The Three Rules to Lose Weight and Keep It Off Forever. This book will teach you how to lose weight without hunger, significant deprivations, counting calories or carbs, or medical intervention. Simply put, we completely avoid certain carbohydrates, what I call bad carbs. Soon, I will explain in more detail what carbohydrates are and which ones should be considered bad. For now, carbohydrates are sugars and molecules we break down into sugars. You'll quickly learn what to avoid and what to eat so you can lose weight and not gain it back. You can do it right away, and you can do it forever.

This book is not for everyone. It isn't for you if you expect an easy solution. You must give up something. You cannot eat everything you like, everything you've eaten that led to you becoming overweight, and yet still lose weight. The economist Thomas Sowell said, "Life does not ask us what we want. It presents us with options." You can lose weight and keep it off, or you can eat everything you want, as much as you want. If you choose the first option, then this book is for you. It will sometimes be challenging. But most people who have ever lived on this planet lived within The Three Rules. They did it out of necessity. Still, if they did it, we can do it. For me, the benefits of weight loss, followed by weight control, are worth the effort. I hope it's the same for you.

I don't want to tell you The Three Rules and leave it at that. I want you to understand the problem of obesity and why we should fight it. Don't be deceived by those who say obesity is okay. Obesity is associated with a shorter life, a worse quality of life, poor mental health, and many medical conditions. Yes, some obese people are content the way they are, but most would admit that they would rather lose weight if they could. You need to know why it is so difficult to manage your weight. Before you adopt The Three Rules, you need to know about other potential solutions to the obesity problem and why these may or may not be for you. Since committing to The Rules is a big step, you must first understand it, why it works, and why it's the best option for most of us.[1] The Three Rules plan and this book are not perfect. As with any rule, there are gray areas. I have minimized them and have explained the few that remain. Don't get hung up on these very few minor issues. If you do, you will miss the larger picture.

Losing weight is always difficult, requiring serious effort and changes in many parts of your daily routine. I will go over some

---

[1] It is time to go over shortcuts and grammar. If I talk about The Three Rules to Lose Weight and Keep It Off Forever, I may refer to it as The Three Rules, The Rules, The Rules to Lose Weight, and so on. I will capitalize "Rules," so it is clear I'm referring to The Three Rules. I like to refer to The Three Rules as singular because The Rules all go together as one single plan, but sometimes it sounds wrong, and I will use the plural. So usually, but not always, it will be "The Three Rules is…" Also, rather than say carbohydrate or carbohydrates over and over, I will usually write carb or carbs.

reasons it's so difficult. It will seem so hard that many of you will not want to put in the effort. But once into the diet for a few weeks, most people realize that while their routines have changed, it isn't as hard as they thought.

The basis of The Three Rules is that certain carbohydrates cause nearly all our weight gain. You don't want a science book, and I haven't given you one. But you need to know how these carbohydrates cause weight gain to understand why you should stop eating some of your favorite foods. I will discuss each Rule in enough detail so there can be no misunderstandings. The Rules work, and they are simple, but some points will need explaining. Losing weight and keeping it off are different mentally; you will learn how to do both. I don't want you to lose weight just to gain it back—it's demoralizing. Some pitfalls can sabotage your plans, and you will learn to avoid them. I will teach you tips that help every minute and every day while you succeed and if or when you slip up.

Most importantly, you will learn how to enjoy life under The Rules. You will improve your health, quality of life, and well-being. As hard as it is to believe, you will love eating, probably more than you do now.

Eating in a way that improves health and controls weight is like accomplishing other life goals. Over the years, I have succeeded and failed at many projects. I've been successful recently with my weight. I've been successful in my career as a physician. For the most part, I have been successful in my family life. But I've failed at many things: projects started and quit, friendships fallen by the wayside, and more than a few family issues. Discipline, focus, and planning have led to my greatest successes. Living by The Three Rules will help you lose weight and keep it off. But eating with intent and thinking about what you eat helps in all aspects of life—we succeed best if we think about what we're doing and do everything with intent.

I know that if you follow The Rules, you will lose weight. If you succeed, then I've accomplished my goal. If the concepts of The Rules help you with other parts of your life, then so much the better. The Three Rules will make most people healthier. But everything has a risk—driving, walking outside, and even taking a shower. There are a few risks of this and any diet plan. Please talk to your doctor to make sure The Three Rules to Lose Weight and Keep It Off Forever is okay for you to start. I hope it is because you will be better for it.

Part 1

The Problem

"It is the truth I seek, and the truth
never harmed anyone."
Marcus Aurelius

People have gotten heavier. If you are my age, you remember that in school, there were a few obese kids and a few obese parents. You would hear people talking about how heavy a particular boy, girl, or parent might be. Now, there are so many overweight and obese people that there isn't much point in mentioning a person's weight as a describing feature.

The current definition of obesity for adults is having a body mass index or BMI (a formula based on the relationship of weight to height) of 30 or higher. Overweight is a BMI of 25 or higher. These are not new or more rigid definitions. The statistics are staggering. In a recent survey by the Centers for Disease Control (CDC), 42% of adults in the United States are obese,[2] and over 70% are overweight or obese. Obesity is so common that what we see all the time, what

---

[2] https://www.cdc.gov/obesity/data/adult.html

we think of as "normal," is now overweight or obese. About 9% of Americans are severely obese, also called morbidly obese, defined as a BMI of 40 or higher. The statistics for children are equally alarming. Obesity in children is a BMI at or above the 95th percentile by standard growth charts. 19.7% of children and adolescents under 20 and 12.7% of children between 2 and 5 years old meet this definition.[3]

We will discuss some reasons for the increase in obesity, but first, I want to go over the harms of obesity and why we should fight it. Some politicians and others talk about obesity's financial burden on society and the health care system. I don't care about that, at least not for this book. I care about you and your health and well-being. You will benefit from knowing the potential harms of being overweight so you can decide if the hard work needed to fight it is worth the effort.

There is a movement to accept obesity. I accept everyone. No one sets out to become obese. No one sets out to get cancer or any other illness. I accept and respect the obese and overweight, just like I accept and respect those with cancer and other diseases. There are ad campaigns showing that obese people are beautiful. Of course, there are beautiful obese people. There are beautiful people with cancer. But I still want to get rid of the cancer.

---

[3] https://www.cdc.gov/obesity/data/childhood.html

Adverse Effects of
Obesity and Why We Should Fight It

*If you don't understand the harms of something,
why would you put in the effort to fight it?*

It's a cliché that you must want to quit something to succeed. That is true, but I don't think it's a helpful or sufficient sentiment. Many or most smokers in their hearts want to quit smoking, and many or most obese people want to lose weight. But that doesn't mean much. To quit smoking or lose weight, you need incentive enough to do it so you can overcome the difficulties. I believe that the vast majority of smokers would quit in an instant if doing so would save the life of a loved one. Many would never smoke again if offered 10 million dollars. If offered the same threat or reward, most obese people would commit to losing weight, whatever the difficulties.

I am not saying that people with a weight problem don't want to lose weight—just the opposite. I believe most do want to lose weight. You would not have bought this book if you didn't want to lose weight. But that is not the point. Do you have enough incentive to make the extreme effort that losing weight requires? It takes effort. But I don't think it's as extreme as it seems. In retrospect, most people who lose weight with The Three Rules believe it wasn't that hard. Looking forward, the effort may seem daunting. Looking back, not so much.

In this chapter, I will give you reasons to make the effort. Some facts are scary, but they are true. The truth does not harm us—the willful ignorance of the truth does.

Health Problems

Does obesity always lead to health problems? No, many healthy people are obese. But that doesn't mean much. There are many healthy smokers, some living into old age. There are healthy people who drink too much alcohol, reckless drivers who have never been hurt, and drunk drivers who have never suffered the consequences. But it's undeniable that obesity increases the risks of many health problems, and I expect you already know most of these risks. Many health issues are especially linked to the pattern of obesity, with visceral or deep fat, the fat in the "apple" or "beer belly" pattern, being the worst, but just being heavy is a problem.

Type 2 diabetes, which used to be called adult-onset diabetes, is seen principally in the overweight and obese. When I graduated medical school in 1992, we didn't see many adult diabetics. We didn't consider this type of diabetes a big deal, and we rarely needed to treat it with insulin. In my practice, I followed hundreds of patients with diabetes, and at least 90% were overweight or obese. There are genetic risks, but weight is the most significant factor. If you don't become overweight, diabetes is unlikely. If you have diabetes and you lose weight, diabetes almost always improves, usually dramatically. As I mentioned in the previous chapter, improvement or remission of diabetes is the rule after weight loss. It's the most important thing. Type 1 diabetics have an absolute requirement for insulin, are not usually overweight, and should talk to their doctor before they attempt a weight loss program.

Type 2 diabetes (I will say diabetes from here on) is associated with other health problems and is a leading cause of premature death. I had patients with diabetes who said they were okay because they controlled their sugars with medications. But that only lowers the risk of certain diabetic complications—it doesn't eliminate them, and it doesn't lower the risk of dying all that much. The best defense against diabetes is to lose weight and keep it off. Studies, too many to count, have shown the benefits of weight loss in diabetes prevention and treatment. It is the very first thing I mentioned to my diabetic patients.

If you are overweight or obese, and you don't have diabetes, you are not off the hook, not even close. Borderline diabetes, sometimes known as prediabetes, also linked to weight, is a serious problem. Many prediabetics have a condition called the metabolic syndrome. Blood glucose is mildly elevated, blood pressure is high, abdominal fat is increased, and cholesterol is abnormal. People with metabolic syndrome often develop diabetes, but even those who don't are at significantly higher risk of heart disease and other problems.

Polycystic ovary disease is an increasingly common condition linked to obesity and diabetes. It can lead to infertility, excessive hair growth, and irregular periods. Weight loss and its benefits on sugar control usually help.

Fatty liver, also called non-alcoholic fatty liver disease, is often diagnosed in overweight and obese people and is uncommon in those with normal weight. Most physicians were unaware of this condition when I was in medical school. In fact, Eugene Schiff, MD, a renowned hepatologist, was my attending in medical school when we made the diagnosis of fatty liver in a non-drinker. It was such a novel disease that we presented it at a conference. When I retired, I was seeing patients with fatty liver every single day, often multiple times. While fatty liver often doesn't lead to ill effects, it is so common in the United States that it's now a leading cause of cirrhosis, a serious, sometimes fatal disease.

Heart disease is far more likely in the obese. Many obese people have normal cholesterol and no heart disease, but remember that there are many risk factors, and obesity is just one. If you are obese, your risk of coronary disease and having a heart attack is higher. The strain that obesity places on the heart can also lead to heart failure, where the heart cannot keep up with demand. The legs swell, and fluid builds up in the lungs. Patients have trouble breathing, and abnormal heart rhythms often develop. Both coronary disease and heart failure can lead to sudden death. When you see a story about a celebrity dying suddenly and they were obese, you're likely not all that surprised.

Blood clots occur more frequently in obese people. These can happen without warning or after major surgery. It is sometimes fatal when the clots go into the lung, a condition called a pulmonary embolism. When I hear of someone dying after surgery, especially if they were obese, I think of a blood clot.

Stroke, devastating damage to the brain caused by a blood clot or bleeding, is directly linked to weight, and reaching a BMI of 30 doubles the risk.[4] Losing weight lowers that risk. Strokes happen in thin people, but we see more and more obese stroke victims yearly. Some say they don't mind dying as long as they can eat whatever they want. Well, stroke often leads to disability and complete dependence on others. I would give up certain foods to lower that risk.

Atrial fibrillation, a common heart rhythm problem, can lead to stroke, heart failure, and other serious problems. The prevalence of atrial fibrillation is increasing, primarily because of obesity. In several impressive studies, weight loss markedly improves the success rate of treatment of atrial fibrillation.[5]

Sleep apnea, an important and sometimes fatal condition where a person doesn't breathe effectively while sleeping, is closely linked to weight, and 90% of sufferers are obese. Sleep apnea causes daytime sleepiness, headaches, mental health issues, and high blood pressure. When I saw an overweight patient with these problems, I ordered a sleep study first.

Arthritis, especially of the knees and hips, causes significant pain and disability and is much more of a problem in the obese. It is well

---

[4] Kurth T, Gaziano JM, Berger K, et al. Body mass index and the risk of stroke in men. Arch Intern Med. 2002;162(22):2557-2562. doi:10.1001/archinte.162.22.2557

[5] Pathak RK, Middeldorp ME, Meredith M, et al. Long-Term Effect of Goal-Directed Weight Management in an Atrial Fibrillation Cohort: A Long-Term Follow-Up Study (LEGACY). J Am Coll Cardiol. 2015;65(20):2159-2169. doi:10.1016/j.jacc.2015.03.002

known and somewhat obvious that if someone puts more weight on damaged joints, it will hurt more, just as my knees hurt more when I carry a bag of water softener salt to the basement. It now seems that obesity can directly cause inflammation in multiple joints, even in the hands.[6] So, obesity makes arthritis both more likely and more painful. Anyone with arthritis understands the effect it has on their quality of life.

Obesity is linked to worse outcomes in respiratory infections. As I proofread this chapter, we are still dealing with the COVID-19 pandemic. It has become clear that obesity is a significant risk factor for severe complications and death from the Coronavirus. Over the next decade, when we look back at what we could have done to prevent more deaths from this infection, we may realize that being in better health would have been the best defense.

You probably already know about some of the medical problems described above, but this may surprise you—it surprised most of my patients. Obesity can cause cancer, and some estimate that excessive weight causes 40% of all cancers.[7] It isn't immediately intuitive, but obesity leads to cancer through inflammation and hormonal changes. Many types of cancer are linked to weight, and for four types, obesity is more of a risk factor than smoking. As the rate of

---

[6] Visser AW, Ioan-Facsinay A, de Mutsert R, et al. Adiposity and hand osteoarthritis: the Netherlands Epidemiology of Obesity study. *Arthritis Res Th er*. 2014;16(1):R19. Published 2014 Jan 22. doi:10.1186/ar4447

[7] Steele CB, Thomas CC, Henley SJ, et al. Vital Signs: Trends in Incidence of Cancers Associated with Overweight and Obesity - United States, 2005-2014. MMWR Morb Mortal Wkly Rep. 2017;66(39):1052-1058. Published 2017 Oct 3. doi:10.15585/mmwr.mm6639e1

smoking falls, obesity may soon overtake tobacco use as the leading preventable risk factor for cancer.

I could go on for many more pages about the health risks of obesity—weight is linked to skin changes, fractures, asthma, neurologic conditions, and many other illnesses. However, some other consequences of obesity may be even more significant, and I will move on to these.

Quality Of Life

Like the physical problems associated with obesity, the non-physical consequences don't affect everyone. Many, perhaps most, people with weight issues are happy. But the fact remains that some overweight and obese people are unhappy because of their weight problems. Depression and anxiety are linked to weight, both as a cause and effect. Depressed and anxious people often eat more, and obesity can cause or worsen depression and anxiety. This can lead to a cycle of guilt and depression, followed by weight gain, leading to more guilt and depression. Although there is a trend toward less fat-shaming, it still occurs. As she explains in her excellent book, *The Willpower Instinct*, Kelly McGonigal details this problem in a way that hits home for many of us.[8] Overweight people may feel ashamed of what others think of them. The irony for many who overeat is that they cannot enjoy eating because of guilt. Many patients told me they feel bad when eating something fattening. They love ice cream, but

---

[8] McGonigal, Kelly. (2012). The Willpower Instinct: How self-control works, why it matters, and what you can do to get more of it. New York, NY, US: Avery/Penguin Group USA.

even in the privacy of their homes, they feel guilty about an indulgence. Again, this guilt can lead to even more eating.

Even without clinical depression, anxiety, or guilt, the quality of life of heavy people is affected. Activities that young, fit people do are much more difficult for the overweight. Before I wrote the first edition, my wife and I had recently spent two weeks in Yellowstone and Grand Teton National Parks. We hiked miles every day and met many people on the trails. A few were overweight. A smaller number were obese. None were morbidly obese.

A few months before I started this edition, we spent two weeks in Yosemite, Sequoia, and Kings Canyon National Parks. We saw heavy people only near the road pull-offs or on flat trails. The uphill trails were usually too steep for them. Our national parks are spectacular vacations for so many people. Yet the best parts of these parks, the trails in the mountains, are virtually off-limits to those with a severe weight problem. The same is true for other active vacations and activities. I don't see many obese people biking or walking the trails in Minnesota. The serenity of nature can be challenging to access for the obese. What do you do if friends or family invite you on a trip or activity you know you can't do? Unfortunately, this often leads to avoiding these activities and losing contact with others. It may seem impossible to imagine, given how your life is now, but it isn't at all unlikely when you get older and perhaps heavier; I saw it all the time in my practice. I hope that if I am lucky enough to have grandchildren, I can go with them and our son on any vacation—of course, I have to be invited first, which is another question entirely.

You may not be interested or worried about the big trips. Maybe you don't care about hiking, biking, or even walking in the park. But since our physical strength worsens as we age, even simple activities will become more difficult. Engaging with your family and friends can be a problem. You may not be able to play with your kids or grandkids. If you can do it now, can you imagine doing so when you're older and heavier? Will you be able to play catch with a grandchild? Will you sled with your nieces (if you're lucky enough to live in Minnesota?) Get in and out of the boat to teach your grandchild to fish? Work in the garden? Many activities will become difficult or impossible. These activities connect us to our families. So many people miss out on life.

I had patients who, because of their weight, could not easily live on their own. Even simple things like getting out of a chair, shopping in the grocery store, and climbing stairs at a ballgame were more difficult. Just watch people. The heavier a person is, the slower and more labored their actions. I had patients who couldn't take their shoes off to show me a foot problem, and I helped them put on their socks. These examples won't apply to many or most of the obese, but you get the idea. There are significant difficulties in being heavy.

We can fight it. You have to want to fight it. You will need to find the reasons to lose weight, and today is the best day to do anything meaningful. Benjamin Franklin said, "Don't put off until tomorrow what you can do today." Start today.

Self-Image

Happy people usually have a good overall image of themselves. They believe that they are friendly and pleasant to be with. They typically feel good about their physical appearance. I want that for everyone. But do happy people have a good self-image because they are happy? Or are they happy because they have a good self-image? It's probably a bit of both.

Despite the media and celebrities telling us that fat is beautiful, many overweight people don't believe it. They may try to believe that they look good, but when they look in the mirror, they're not pleased. Again, this isn't a rule, and it may not even be true for most people, but it's true for some. I only mention body self-image to give you one more incentive to fight obesity and make a serious effort to lose weight. Self-image shouldn't be the only reason you lose weight, but if it helps you, all the better. If you don't have important reasons to lose weight, you will not make the effort, and you will fail. Everyone who loses weight feels better physically, and everyone who loses weight feels better about themselves.

Why Do People Become Obese?

Only humans, our pets, and our domesticated animals are obese. All other animals fight for their lives to get enough food.

In the distant past, humans had to eat what they could get to survive. Like other animals in the wild, we ate nearly everything we came across that wasn't poisonous. Not long ago, it was said that we had to work to feed our families. Now, far from starving, even the poor in this country are obese. That is a testament to the overall wealth of the United States and most of the developed world. With a modest salary, the price of food isn't much of a factor in our caloric intake. We have plentiful, high-energy food, providing much more than we need. Yet we still eat as if we will never find food again. We don't worry about our next meal, and we keep eating. I call that eating without intent. We don't consciously think about what we eat. When we buy things without intent, we go into debt. When we eat without intent, we gain weight.

On the other side of the energy equation, we use much less. Think about how much physical effort it took a hundred years ago to manage your home and life. People burned significant calories in their daily lives by washing and drying clothes by hand, using a heavy, old-fashioned iron, pushing a non-powered lawnmower, cleaning floors, and building a fire. Now, people think they're active when they walk a few thousand steps at the office. No wonder it takes genuine effort to avoid gaining weight in the modern world. That would have been a laughable statement when our great-grandparents were born.

In the clinic, someone who had gained weight often asked me to test them for a slow metabolism or thyroid problem. They told me they were eating the same as they used to and had gained weight. But if you're not measuring food, counting the times you eat out, and counting all the calories you burn, you don't know that you're doing everything the same. Some say they eat what their friends eat but gain more weight than their friends. But you don't see what your friends do when you're not with them. You may go out to dinner more than they do. You may get the large fries, and they get the small. They may skip meals or exercise more.

If it's so easy to gain weight, why are there any thin people? Most thin people today work at it. They rarely eat junk food, or they may frequently diet. We think they're not fighting obesity, but we don't notice what they do to stay fit. We may see them eat junk food occasionally. But for them, it's a treat; for us, it's a habit. They eat at restaurants and eat junk food with us but eat differently when we don't see them. We may eat junk food at home, but they don't. Most of these fit people also exercise—a lot.

There are a few perpetually thin people who don't work at it. These people rarely overeat junk food and never have second helpings. They seldom, if ever, have the urge to eat the things that cause weight gain. I believe these people have a smaller appetite that is inborn or learned at a young age. Some don't crave sweets like other people. We're different, and they have an advantage over us in this aspect of their lives. They may have disadvantages, like motion sickness, migraines, or cravings for something else, like alcohol. We can't worry about people who are perpetually thin or better than us in other ways. We can't worry about the reasons they are the way they are. We have our problems, and they have theirs.

Most people have trouble maintaining a healthy weight. We see it all around us. I want you to understand why and how we can fight it. It is an effort, but you can do it. We cannot continue to do what we're doing and expect our lives to improve. The world will not change for us.

Carbohydrates Are the Most Important

In nature, animals struggle to get enough food. Most of the time, animals use energy as soon as they eat it. When food is more plentiful, the energy is stored as fat for later needs. Since food is usually scarce, animals in the wild rarely get enough food to store fat so they don't become obese. People, until recently, were no exception; only a century ago, starvation was common, even in the United States. Like other animals, we developed a robust system for holding on to almost all the energy we eat, burning as little fuel as possible, and eating as much as possible because days might go by when there would be insufficient food. Now, we have much more food than we need. We don't go days without eating, and many don't go hours. Our portions are larger, we eat more often, and the foods we eat are much more calorie-dense. A single bottle of cola has the calories of three apples. A medium Frappuccino (basically a milkshake) has the calories of five apples.

What has changed the most in our diet over the last few hundred years is our carbohydrate consumption. Our total food intake has increased, but less dramatically than carbohydrates, especially sugar and refined carbs like bread and bread-based products. Carbohydrates are the principal reason behind our obesity problem.

There are three categories of food: carbohydrates, fat, and protein. Carbohydrates are sugars and complex molecules, such as starch, that our bodies convert to sugar. Sugars include **glucose,** which our body uses directly for energy; sucrose or table sugar; fructose from fruit; and lactose, in milk and dairy products. The various sugars have different effects on our metabolism. Multiple sources report that the average American eats 100-150 pounds of sugar yearly, mostly in soft drinks, desserts, and other processed and prepared foods. In 1700, sugar intake was under ten pounds per year. Our intake of starches has also increased, though not to the same extent as sugar.

Fats are found in plants and animals, mainly acting as storage for long-term energy use. Plant fats, except for coconut and palm oils, are liquids and include olive, peanut, and my new favorite, avocado. Most animal fats are solid at room temperature, and we all have seen the fat in steak and bacon. Fats are high in calories, containing nine calories for every gram, while protein and carbohydrates have four calories per gram.

Protein is essential in our diets, with animals being the most significant source. Meat is mostly protein, with varying amounts of fat and minimal if any, carbohydrates. Plants also provide some protein, with the densest source being seeds.

Carbohydrates are the key to the obesity problem. Some carbohydrates, especially sugar, make fat storage easier and more efficient. Nowadays, too much of our diet consists of carbohydrates, especially the types that most contribute to obesity. Over time, nature favored humans who could more easily gain weight, so we began to enjoy sugar and carbs, much like addictive substances. I have never had a problem with addiction to chicken, fish, steak, or other meats and have never been hooked on olive oil. But I have had habit problems with snack foods, bread, candy, pastries, and other high-carb foods. We eat carbs because we like them and can't stop once we start.

When we eat and digest food, the glucose level in our blood rises. We use the glucose we need and store extra energy in the form of fat and glycogen, a complex carbohydrate. As glucose levels increase, insulin levels also increase, allowing for efficient fat storage. Since we are always using energy, we burn fat if we are not storing it. So, even without exercise, we will often be in a negative energy balance, meaning we burn more fat than we make. When we overeat carbs, that doesn't happen; it's more difficult to burn fat and easier to put it on.

When plants are scarce, humans can survive without carbs, making glucose from protein (with a small contribution from fat).

Diets such as the ketogenic diet allow so little carbohydrate that our body enters ketosis, a process seen in starvation. In this state, we make ketones, compounds that our brain can use for energy instead of glucose. The ketogenic diet was around long before the obesity problem took off, used in children for refractory seizures. People on these restrictive diets do not waste away, but they don't become overweight. I will expand on the ketogenic diet later in this book—it can help with weight loss, but most people don't use the term correctly, and partial adherence to the diet can ruin your weight loss plans.

As you will see later, very low-carb diets cause weight loss, even though you can eat virtually as much protein and fat as you want. Ironically, what we have historically thought of as fattening, say a cheeseburger, is fattening more from the carbohydrates in the bread than the calories in the meat and cheese. Peanut butter and jelly sandwiches are fattening because of the bread and jelly, not the high-calorie, high-fat peanut butter unless there is added sugar in it.

Because carbohydrates make fat storage easier, managing carbohydrate consumption is the key to losing weight and the basis of The Three Rules to Lose Weight. Can you eat some carbohydrates on The Three Rules? Absolutely. I eat almost all varieties of fruit and vegetables, nuts, peanuts, beans, whole grains, and dairy.[9] And I eat a lot of it—at least a cup of nuts a day, 2-3 pieces of fruit, lots of cheese and yogurt, and a vast amount of vegetables. My pressure cooker gets

---

[9] We will talk much more about grains since they have variable effects. Refined grains and all rice are against The Rules. There is more to follow, so don't worry about it now.

a workout with all the beans we eat. And remember, since protein and fat matter little to weight gain (if, and only if, you obey the Three Rules), I eat them every day. That includes meat, chicken, fish, cheese, oil, eggs, and nuts.

So why does The Rules plan allow some carbohydrates but not others? Not all carbohydrates raise our blood glucose in the same manner. Since the glucose rise varies by the type of carbohydrate eaten, the efficiency of fat storage also varies. The Three Rules allows you to eat carbohydrates that don't cause a dramatic rise in glucose. What makes The Rules different from other diets is that you don't need to memorize lists of carbohydrates you can eat.

The glycemic index is a medical term that describes how much the glucose level rises after eating. Briefly, if you eat a food sample containing fifty grams of carbohydrates, your glucose will rise a predictable amount.[10] If you eat pure glucose, that rise is defined as one hundred, the highest you can get. Proteins and fats do not have any carbohydrates, so they don't raise blood sugar much, if at all—their glycemic index is zero. Not all foods have been tested, but generalizations are possible based on the index of similar foods. You may read that certain mixtures of food result in a different glycemic index than eating them individually, but that effect is usually small enough that we can ignore it. The higher the glycemic index, the more likely it will cause weight gain.

An additional point worth mentioning is serving size. We all know candy bars are probably not good to eat if you want to lose

---

[10] https://www.gisymbol.com/how-is-gi-measured/

weight. (That is more from the sugar than the fat or the calories.) But what if you had one small square of a candy bar rather than the entire bar? That would be better. But as I will discuss later in the book, most people can't stick to a tiny square. Remember that the glycemic index reflects a fixed fifty-gram amount of carbohydrates. The term **glycemic load** takes into account the serving size. I won't belabor this point, though many diet books do. Some foods, like carrots, have a moderate to high glycemic index. But a carrot has so little total carbohydrate content that you would have to eat many carrots to reach that fifty-gram amount. So, carrots are fine. No one eats so many carrots at one time that it makes a difference.

Conversely, spaghetti is only moderately high on the glycemic index, but typical dry spaghetti in the box has almost fifty grams of carbohydrates in one serving. The serving size is two ounces, one-eighth of a package. When I used to eat spaghetti, I would split a box at most three ways. That is over 2.5 servings each. It is inconceivable to have a spaghetti dinner with one-eighth of a box of spaghetti. Fortunately, The Three Rules doesn't worry too much about serving size, as long as you are not ridiculous, like eating two pounds of carrots at a time.

What about sugar itself? Sugar is the worst thing to eat if you want to lose weight and keep it off. In nature, there isn't much sugar to be eaten. Fruits and vegetables have some, but unless you eat a ton of fruit, there isn't enough sugar to make people obese. Honey is basically liquid table sugar. Honey isn't allowed on The Three Rules, but I doubt anyone got fat on honey because few people are gorging on it.

In the modern world, sugar added to food is the biggest problem. Foods with significant added sugar have a high glycemic index and glycemic load, leading to efficient fat production. In his superb book, *The Case Against Sugar,*[11] Gary Taubes compellingly presents the argument that sugar is the root cause of obesity and many other serious medical problems in the United States, including diabetes, heart disease, and cancer. The Three Rules eliminates added sugar and other problematic carbohydrates in a plan that is simple to follow.

We Don't Make Our Own Food

I am 55 years old. When I was a kid, we didn't eat out much. We made something quick for breakfast and usually packed lunch. We didn't have snack time at school, though sometimes we ate an apple. There was no takeout, and we rarely bought packaged or pre-made meals at the grocery store. Think about your typical week and what kids eat at school. How many meals do you eat at a restaurant, or from takeout or delivery? How many store-bought snacks do you eat? When you go to the gas station, do you get food? When I was young, there was only gas at a gas station.

On average, one-third of people in the United States eat fast food on a given day.[12] Some eat less than that, and some eat more, but that is a lot. And many restaurants and takeout, which don't count toward

---

[11] Taubes, Gary. The Case Against Sugar. First edition. New York: Alfred A. Knopf, 2016.

[12] https://www.cdc.gov/nchs/data/databriefs/db322-h.pdf

that statistic, are worse than fast food. Several Panera Bread sandwiches have more calories and carbs than a Big Mac.

Why does this matter? The calories and carbohydrates in a restaurant are double or even triple that of a home-cooked meal. Restaurants want everything to taste better than what you make at home, so they add butter, sugar, (and salt) at higher levels than you do. The portions are bigger because they want you to think you're getting a good deal. Understandably, they don't care about your diet plan or your goals.

I hear several days a week that eating at home is more expensive than eating out. That's not true. My wife and I will often share a half-chicken. Two chickens at Costco cost about fourteen dollars (even with the recent inflation). That's seven dollars a chicken or $3.50 a half-chicken. I eat half of that for dinner—$1.75. Suppose I eat a half-pound of roasted Brussels sprouts or green beans (a large serving for either) that is at most another $1.50. Frozen vegetables are even less expensive. So, my meal is under $3.50. Few restaurants will cost you less than that. I don't even want to mention how cheap our soup night is. People say eating out is more convenient. Again, I don't believe it. I can make that chicken and vegetable dinner with a few minutes of preparation and then oven time. I can read, watch the news, talk to my wife or son, and so on. I don't have to drive to the restaurant, order, wait for the food, then the check, or drive home. I enjoy eating out, and I do eat out, but I don't do it to be healthier, to spend less money, or to save time.

You can lose weight with The Rules and still eat at restaurants, but you must be more careful. Restaurant chefs only care that your food tastes good and fills you up. It can be high in sugar, other carbs, and salt, though salt isn't relevant for weight control. You may not know precisely what is in the food you get, and they may not even tell you the truth if you ask. Controlling your diet is easier at home.

Making more meals yourself will help you follow The Rules, save money, and save time. You will have more relaxing and meaningful conversations with friends and family. Preparing meals and eating at home with my family are important parts of my life, adding immensely to my happiness. I strongly recommend it.

We Get Little Exercise

I asked most of my patients if they exercised. Thankfully, some exercised regularly, but a majority told me that while they didn't do formal exercise, they were active all day. I don't know what that means. They told me they were up and down all the time, cleaning, mowing the lawn, and so on. None of those activities is what I mean by exercise. Mowing the lawn or playing golf burns more calories and does more good for your health than sitting on the couch eating bonbons, as my mother used to say. But compare this description of being active to what everyone did only fifty or a hundred years ago.

People a hundred years ago burned far more calories than we do; we live a life of luxury by comparison. Most homes in the United States have dishwashers, washing machines, dryers, vacuum cleaners, electric irons, and on and on. Doing the laundry used to be a grueling, full-day chore—chopping wood, feeding the stove, heating the water, scrubbing the clothes, putting the clothes on the clothesline, folding, and probably other steps I don't even know about. Not that I iron my clothes now, but if you have ever picked up an old iron, you know how heavy they are. You had to heat the iron repeatedly over the stove and slide the iron carefully on the clothes until the iron cooled. Then, you took a second iron off the stove and replaced it with the cool iron. It was laborious and burned many calories. What we take for granted today as a minor task was difficult work back then. It's easy to understand why most people were lean. You couldn't easily become obese with their diet and that level of exertion. If you ever became short on food, you lost weight.

In the past, usually only the wealthy would become overweight—regular people were thin, and poor people starved. Only the rich had enough food to gain weight in significant amounts. Poor people today are not thin or wasting away, at least not in the United States or other developed countries. In fact, the poor are more often overweight than the wealthy. Even poor people have electric or gas heating, laundry machines or access to a laundromat, and other modern tools to maintain the home. We have cars or public transportation, seldom walking any significant distance anywhere. In the past, the wealthy were sometimes overweight because they could afford rich foods and had thin servants to do the work and drive them places in their horse-drawn carriages. Daily work requires much less energy now, and we all have access to effort-saving tools that didn't exist a hundred years ago.

Exercise is not one of the Three Rules to Lose Weight, but it's important. Exercise burns calories and, therefore, fat. It's good for the heart, helps with stress relief, lowers the risk of multiple medical problems, and gives us a sense of accomplishment. Exercise helps us make the right food choices. I would feel foolish spending an hour on the treadmill and then having a bowl of ice cream. You don't need to exercise to lose weight, but it helps. There is no significant downside to exercise.

We Have Some Bad Habits

A habit is something we do without thinking about it. Some habits are harmless to our health, like cracking knuckles, humming to ourselves, and checking our smartphones, while others are serious and life-threatening, like smoking and drinking. I want to concentrate on the habits ingrained in our lives that contribute to weight gain.

The main issue with our habits is the mindset they create. Our habits reflect our thoughts on health and eating. If a person has a habit of taking the elevator one flight to their office and parking at the nearest spot to the front door, they may also be more likely to eat a muffin at Starbucks every morning rather than an apple at home.

Many of our eating habits can be changed by just paying attention and doing things with intent. They don't require psychologists or medical interventions to break. Stopping at the coffee shop on the way to work isn't subconscious or addictive, but I doubt many people think it through. It's obvious that eating a scone or muffin every morning is worse for our weight than eating a piece of fruit and that a caffè mocha has more calories than coffee and milk. But we don't think about it and keep doing it. Most people think little about the time and money spent every morning they stop for coffee. I would expect this habit could be broken if people added up the five dollars and 15 minutes a day that they spend several days a week.

Similar habits are stopping at a vending machine on the way to your car, buying food at a gas station on the way home from work, grabbing samples at Costco, going to the snack drawer when you get home, and having dessert with dinner. We don't think about all the snacks we put out to watch a football game or the candy and cookies that are everywhere during the holidays, and we don't consider the ice cream we have as a treat nearly every night. A daily treat is just a habit that can be broken by simply becoming aware of it. That is acting with intent.

Being active and exercising is a habit we can start just as easily. The concept of exercise and exertion has changed dramatically over the last hundred years. People only walk places if they live in a big city. When I walk with friends to a restaurant or event, the limit for how far we will walk has shrunk. We automatically drive if it's further than a few blocks. The mindset used to be to walk, but now it's to drive. This isn't a subconscious decision, but we certainly don't think it through. In addition to exercising, a mile walk to lunch is relaxing, gives you time with a friend, avoids the need to find parking or pay for it, and gives you a sense of accomplishment. It is a habit when we do something without thinking about it. The first step to changing the habit is to decide if it's something you want to change.

Taking the elevator instead of stairs is another one. I know this habit is prevalent because it's uncommon for me to meet anyone in the stairwell of any building. If you think it through, the only negative of taking the stairs is the effort. Taking the stairs is quieter, usually faster because you don't have to wait for the elevator, and it's invigorating, especially in the morning. Again, it gives you a sense of accomplishment, and when we feel good about ourselves, we are more likely to do other things that are good for us, such as eating better. My colleagues mocked me for my phobia of germs, but taking the stairs rather than the elevator avoids exposure to viruses, which is especially important during flu season (and, recently, the COVID-19 pandemic). People and websites will tell you that taking the stairs burns only a few calories. That's like saying there are only a few calories in a peanut M and M. Calories and energy add up for better and for worse. But that also ignores the other benefits. I want to develop healthy habits, regardless of the relative contribution of any individual habit.

There are many habits, such as drinking alcohol, that may require outside help to manage. The ones I'm talking about are not that type, though I recommend that everyone who habitually drinks alcohol consider quitting. Doing more activities with intent, with knowledge of the benefits and harms, is very helpful. Think it through. Are there negative consequences to buying snacks, stopping for a Frappuccino and a donut, or taking the elevator? Is this a habit I can change? Just a few minutes of thought leads to profound realizations.

It Is Hard to Lose Weight

"If wishes were fishes, we would all cast nets."
Frank Herbert in Dune

It makes sense that if it is so easy to gain weight, it's even more challenging to lose weight. Ads bombard us on television and the internet about effortless ways to lose weight. They are wrong. There are no easy ways. None. It is rare to achieve any meaningful goal in life by an easy route. Weight loss is no exception. Either accept that it's hard or fail in your attempts. I believe The Three Rules is the best way for most people to lose weight. Like all methods, it is hard, but it's easier in the long run than the other plans. I have tried and have had some success with many diets. They are all difficult, and generally, they all can be effective. Everything we do is a balance between the benefits and the downsides. As hard as The Three Rules can be for some people, the benefits outweigh these difficulties.

Our Bodies Want to Hold on to Fat

For the same reasons we gain weight, it's difficult to lose it. Our bodies are a product of millions of years of evolution. The world has been harsh on all beings, including humans, until recently. We struggled to get enough food, and when we did eat enough, our bodies stored any excess energy immediately, primarily as fat, so we could use it later.

Just like animals that hibernate, we store fat for the times when we don't have enough food. Since lack of food was common in the past, the efficient storage of fat helped us immensely. We might go days without nourishment, certainly many hours, something not very common nowadays. That leaves us with extra fat and no lean times to burn it. Since we don't exercise as much as we used to and eat more than we used to, we have a lot of extra fat.

What happens when we starve ourselves because we are stranded on a desert island, or we cut back intentionally? The same forces for survival want us to keep the fat as long as possible because starvation could last a while. We need energy so we burn fat and lose weight. At least initially, most of the weight loss is fat. Later, we also break down muscle, a downside of starvation diets. Soon, our body adjusts to the calorie cut, slowing our metabolism. That makes the total weight loss less than what would have been predicted. When we eat again in regular quantities, that slow metabolism allows us to gain weight quickly, a helpful trick in the past when food was scarce—not so good now when food is everywhere.

Our bodies fight weight loss, and so do our minds. Evolution gave us a tremendous appetite. Nature designed us to eat *more* than we need for immediate energy use. It's as if we knew we would have periods with inadequate food. We can eat, and we often do eat, whenever food is around. Thousands of years ago, humans couldn't afford to say, "I don't need to eat that apple or fig or leg of deer; I will eat something later." There may have been no food later. We could say that now, but our brain still thinks we shouldn't wait, so we feel hungry and have cravings. This is why your pet Schnoodle will never turn down a treat. Hunger kicks in early in the dieting process, at least in low-calorie diets, long before you lose weight. You must fight the urge to eat for a long time before you even start losing weight. Since your body adjusts to the lower food intake, you continue to be hungry through the entire dieting process. It is difficult to fight a primal urge like hunger. When I used to lose weight by cutting calories, I knew the scale was unlikely to show weight loss if I didn't wake up hungry.

Through various metabolic mechanisms, our bodies want us to hold on to all our fat. Our appetite wants to prevent starvation. As we learned in the last chapter, the types of foods that are constantly around us make it easy to put fat right back on.

Times Have Changed

In the not-too-distant past, it was easier to lose weight because of our more difficult lives. You had to work hard to get enough food to keep weight on. Times have changed in the United States and most of the modern world. As a percentage of our wages, food is much cheaper. Healthy food or junk food, it doesn't matter. You can get chicken for a couple of dollars a pound. On the Walmart website, a two-serving frozen pizza is listed for $3.36, and we have high inflation right now. A ten-serving package of hot dogs is $2.84. A twenty-serving bag of rice is $1.77. If you make ten dollars an hour, you can feed your family on an hour's wages for a day or two. Since most of you reading this book make over ten dollars an hour, you may not even have to consider the cost of the food you and your family eat.

Food is also much more available. If you live in a city, there is food at virtually every corner. On my six-mile drive to work, I traveled one major street. There are over twenty food establishments, at least ten of which are fast food, and I'm not counting five coffee shops. I recently read a Dickens book set in the 1800s, and even the wealthy had just a few options for finding food in an entire small town.

You used to buy groceries at the grocery store to make meals at home from scratch. Now, you can purchase all kinds of ready-made foods. The bakery section at the new monster store near my house is bigger than entire markets of old. Premade meals are so prevalent that stores have a new name: "grocerants." Premade meals are usually more expensive than preparing meals yourself, but they are still inexpensive compared to the cost of food in the past. Junk food is cheap.

The grocery store has healthy food in the produce aisles, the sections often labeled "healthy," and the meat and seafood areas. But the areas devoted to less healthy options have expanded. I love grocery shopping, so my wife seldom sees the inside of a store. She was recently surprised that the frozen potato section is an entire aisle, and the other frozen vegetables fit in one or two freezers. There is far more ice cream than health food by a wide margin. There is more candy than beans, cookies than olive oil, cereal than yogurt, potato chips than hummus—you get the picture.

You don't need to buy ice cream, prepared meals, pies, or candy, and no one is forcing you to eat it. But the more you see something, the more you'll think it's normal and acceptable to eat it, and the more you will be tempted by it. I always struggle to say no, so I try not to get exposed to temptations. No wonder patients ask me, "What do you eat?" when I tell them I don't eat what I call junk food. Junk is all they see when they shop. Here, also, I use the analogy of alcohol—a recovering alcoholic should probably avoid bars and liquor stores, where every choice is alcohol.

Time is more of a factor today. We know that cooking at home is healthier and usually less expensive. But with so many distractions and other activities, managing our time requires significant effort. We know exercise is good for us, but we can't find time for it either. Before smartphones, hundreds of television channels, streaming, and social media, we had less to do. Now, many of these distractions have become necessities. We think we have little time to cook or exercise, and sometimes it's true, but we probably could carve out 45 minutes to prepare a simple meal and exercise. It has become increasingly difficult to focus on these tasks with so much going on. Fortunately, The Three Rules requires only a few minutes to prepare a simple meal or a few seconds at a restaurant to choose something healthy.

Our Minds Make It Harder

We tell ourselves things that make it harder to lose weight. This may once have been a helpful instinct to get us to eat as much as possible, but it's not beneficial now when we rarely have a food shortage. Our minds do the same thing with every habit, but changing our diet is harder because food is everywhere. Again, a superb source for this aspect of losing weight is *The Willpower Instinct*.

Procrastination is the enemy of success in all things. In school, kids will do anything to avoid starting a project. The same is true for changing habits. Is there a good reason not to eat better right now? Why do we have to wait until tomorrow to avoid fast food? Is Thursday a better day to eat right? Or to exercise? Yet we all do it. We say we'll eat better tomorrow because today we're going out with Jane and John. Or I don't have time to cook today. Or Teddy has baseball practice after school.

Again, I use the analogy of alcohol or drug addiction. With a friend who is an alcoholic, would you advise them to quit alcohol tomorrow? "Tonight, drink up; tomorrow is an outstanding day to quit." It sounds silly. But we say that to ourselves with food. "Tonight, I'll enjoy the burger and fries and start eating better tomorrow." But tomorrow, there is something else to delay the start.

When we eventually start a plan to lose weight, our minds sabotage us. We make up reasons we need the cookie or the doughnut. We license ourselves to eat when we know we shouldn't. People in my office ran to get the free ice cream someone brought for Nurses' Week. We wouldn't usually eat ice cream at 10:00 a.m., but we had to—it's Nurses' Week. In early January, people blamed their weight gain on holiday treats at the office. So, a 50-cent cookie is okay to eat if it's free? If it were a rare event, that wouldn't be a problem. But it isn't a rare event. Treats can become almost a daily occurrence, and a daily treat is just a habit. You must stick to any diet, even The Three Rules, for it to work. We have all said, "I know I shouldn't do it, but just this once." We know what happens next.

Our minds tell us it's okay to go off a diet because it's a holiday or a vacation. Why we should ruin our diet on vacation, I don't understand. A recovering alcoholic knows not to drink alcohol on vacation. And no one should cheat on their spouse because they're on vacation. So why would we cheat on our diet? But we do. A vacation is still our life. If something is worthwhile, we should do it on vacation. But our minds tell us otherwise.

We are also likely to go off our diet when we're upset or something bad happens. Yes, getting in a fight with someone at work is upsetting. But it has nothing to do with a Big Mac and fries at McDonald's. Yet our minds make us think eating at McDonald's will decrease our anger at a colleague. The relationship between mood and eating is probably universal.

When a good thing happens, our minds also tell us it's okay to eat off our plan. We get a raise, so we can have chicken wings. Our boss praises us, and it's ice cream all around. Logically, when something good happens at work, we should improve ourselves. Yet our minds tell us otherwise, and we give ourselves the false reward of unhealthy eating.

Injuries can be even more mind-altering. I've never counted, but I estimate that three times a week, a patient of mine told me they had gained weight because of an injury. Perhaps they had sprained an ankle five weeks before, and that explained their six-pound weight gain. Why they couldn't lift weights, do push-ups, slowly walk, or even bike, I can't explain. Why an ankle sprain caused them to drink a

Frappuccino or eat an ice cream sundae at Costco was unexplained. But we all play these mind tricks, hurting only ourselves.

Even when we are trying to eat better, we fool ourselves. Last year, a study was published in *Circulation* looking at the perception of diet quality in people trying to lose weight.[13] A hundred people were told to improve their diet and report on it. Their assessment was compared to the assessment of nutritionists. According to the authors, "the majority of participants appear to perceive their diet quality and improvements in diet quality as better than measured." I've seen this same pattern with exercise. Many think of ten thousand steps gathered during a typical workday (and most devices count small steps) as exercise. I suppose it is, but it isn't the same as a 40-minute power walk.

Logically, we know we should eat better starting today. We know we should exercise starting today. We know that fighting with a friend shouldn't lead to unhealthy eating. Then why do we do what we do? Since eating and relaxing are so pleasant in the short term, our subconscious wants that pleasure to offset the pain or increase the joy of the situation. But we are logical, rational beings. To succeed in any diet plan or any meaningful endeavor, we must overcome these natural urges. We can follow The Rules at all times, good or bad, on vacation or at work, in restaurants or at home.

---

[13] Cheng J, Costacou T, Rockette-Wagner B, et al. Perceived and calculated diet quality improvements in a randomized mHealth weight loss trial [published online ahead of print, 2023 Feb 15]. Behav Med. 2023;1-6. doi:10.1080/08964289.2023.2178374

With certain patients, I brought up another difficulty in losing weight. I mention it here, knowing many of you will think I'm wrong. Fine, feel free to ignore it and move on. Recently, we've developed a different concept of hard work. So many of us, and I have sometimes been guilty, are unwilling to work as hard at something as is necessary. It isn't easy to lose weight. Do it anyway. If a child tells a parent that the homework is hard, perhaps the proper response is, "Do it anyway." Ryan Holiday's books, especially *The Obstacle Is the Way*, reminded me of this critical fact. Difficulty shouldn't stop us. It should lead us to be better. Yes, it was hard for me to lose weight. It's hard to keep it off. With The Rules, I am doing it anyway.

Other People Make It Harder

You want to lose weight. Your friends and family would, if pressed, agree that you should lose weight. Yet the people around you often make it more difficult. Occasionally, people secretly want us to remain overweight—perhaps to make themselves feel better. This malice is rare, and their interference in weight loss is usually unintentional. Everyone has problems that they can't solve easily. When we see someone succeed, we feel a little insecure about ourselves, wondering why we can't be successful. When our friend gets a new job, we feel happy for them, but it's tinged with envy. If a friend gets married, we might be a little jealous. And when someone works hard and loses weight, jealousy can be there. Even without such thoughts, the people we know can make it difficult. They won't be participating in your diet plan, continuing to eat whatever they want.

You may have issues at home if you have a family or a roommate. You may want to eat better, yet your spouse keeps chocolate chip cookies in the pantry. Your son comes home from college and needs to buy a box of Twinkies to roast at the fire pit. (I'm told they are better than s'mores.) Your roommate orders pizza, but you want something healthy. It's hard enough to eat right when it is just you. Like at a grocery store, you may cave in if you're tempted enough times.

Work is even more challenging. Office colleagues bring treats. When you decline, they say, "One Christmas cookie won't kill you." True—one cookie won't kill you. But can you stop at one? Even one cookie could negate your diet successes of the day. These people don't mean to sabotage your diet, but it happens all too often. At the end of a workday, you plan to go to the gym, but a friend asks you to go out for a drink. Even if you tell them about your exercise and weight loss plans and they say they understand, you can see the disappointment on their face. How often will you go out with them instead of the gym?

When you have lost some weight, even a lot of weight, other things happen. Your friends may say how good you look and comment on your discipline, but with a subtle comment like, "I could never give up my bagel and cream cheese." Or "Don't you like beer?" These comments remind us of things we've given up to accomplish our goals. I don't entirely understand the psychology, but I suspect these people can justify their inability to give up certain foods or commit to a goal by pointing out what you are missing out on. I heard similar comments when I studied instead of partied in college.

You must understand and fight the challenges to succeed in weight loss or with any significant goal. Say "no" to people offering treats—it won't offend them. If it does, it tells you a lot about them. Tell your roommate you want to get something other than pizza; you may have to tell your son to keep Twinkies out of the house. Stick to your plans, regardless of the distractions.

It Is Hard to Keep Weight Off

It is demoralizing to work for a year to lose weight, only to gain it back in a month or two.

In my struggles, I have gained as much weight as I have lost, except for the last time. The last time I lost weight, I stuck to The Rules and have kept it off since. I've lost about 550 pounds and gained about 520 pounds, and the weight gain was twice as fast. Remember, our bodies want us to gain weight and store energy for the times when there is inadequate food.

This is a brief chapter. We've already discussed why we become overweight and why it's hard to lose weight. The reasons it's hard to keep weight off are much the same, and we gain the weight back the same way we gained it in the first place. But why do we gain it back so quickly? And if we've put in all that effort to lose weight, why do we waste that struggle and gain the weight back anyway?

Some reasons for gaining weight back quickly are physical, such as metabolism changes, but most are mental. It usually comes down to a loss of focus on the problem. We don't pay attention to our diet at the same level as we did when trying to lose weight. We think we don't need to work as hard. In many ways, keeping weight off takes more attention and effort than losing weight.

We Do Not Have a Plan

Most diets, such as the Atkins Diet and Weight Watchers, are designed solely for weight loss. The diets may have maintenance programs, but these are usually vague and less intensive. I don't know too many people who are strict adherents to the maintenance stage of any regimented diet. Most people abandon their diet, returning to their previous lives and habits.

About ten times a day, I discussed weight with patients. Some of them scheduled their appointment to coincide with the start of a diet. This was especially common in January with New Year's resolutions. They talked about The Whole 30, the ketogenic diet, the paleo diet, whatever. I encouraged them and offered a little guidance. But I always asked them what they planned to do after losing weight. Most of the time, they'd given it little thought. At best, they said they hoped to make it a lifestyle change rather than a diet (a common cliché and effective but rarely enacted). They hoped to stay on the maintenance phase of the diet forever, but it seldom worked out that way. If they lost the weight, life got in the way, and they didn't stay on the maintenance plan. They may have had a plan, but when the time came, it fell apart.

The key is to find a plan that works during the diet phase and after, a plan that you can stick to forever, a strategy that can handle life and its inevitable challenges. You need a simple system to eat with intent, thinking about what you are doing at all times.

Our Bodies Adjust to Our Diet

Historically, we would lose weight by eating less, mainly unintentionally, when the food supply was limited. Now, we only eat less if we're trying to watch our weight. Our bodies do not want us to lose weight because if we do, we won't have enough reserve to survive times of inadequate food. If our weight is stable when we eat 2000 calories a day, we will lose some weight when we cut our daily calorie intake to 1500. But over the next few months, our metabolism slows, and we burn less than 2000, maybe only 1600 calories daily. Our weight loss slows, then stalls, and we give up. If we reach our goal for weight loss, we usually go back to eating the 2000 calories again (or more).

But now, we're no longer stable at 2000 calories per day; since our bodies only need 1600 calories, we gain weight. Eventually, that stops as our metabolism reestablishes its 2000 calorie per day requirement. By then, we will have gained at least some of our hard-lost weight back. You will gain even more if you eat over 2000 calories per day.

Fortunately, The Three Rules and other carbohydrate-based plans have less of a problem in this regard. Weight loss can slow down, but less so than the low-calorie diets. The Three Rules are meant to be followed indefinitely, so even if your body adjusts and weight loss slows, it doesn't matter. You are unlikely ever to gain your weight back.

You may wonder why anyone would follow The Three Rules when they don't follow other diet plans. The Rules are different; they are simple and easy to follow. You give up some foods, but there is so much you can eat and enjoy that there is no reason to quit.

We Lose Focus

In anything, it is difficult to sustain focus long term. We throw ourselves into a project, paying attention to all the little details. After a while, we lose that intensity. We see this in sports when a team wins at the beginning of the season only to fall off in the home stretch. Students make careless errors at the end of a long exam. Dieting can be a lengthy process, but keeping the weight off is forever. You may watch everything you eat for a few months, even a year. Then you stop reading labels, asking people what's in the food they're giving you, and making healthy meals. A few bad days can lead to weight gain, at least a little. Then, you get discouraged and give up. This is especially common in diets that cause hunger. (Fortunately, The Rules isn't such a diet.) When you're hungry, it's easy to get distracted and eat whatever is near you.

A theme in this book (and a helpful concept in life) is to eat and do everything with intent. I keep that thought in my head most of the time. Do I skip a workout today? What will happen if I eat this cookie? Do I need it? If I don't work out, at least I've thought about it, understanding the consequences of the decision. Suppose I want to eat the cookie despite the consequences. Fine, I eat the cookie with intent, focusing on what I am doing. This is an excellent way to think about even minor day-to-day decisions. We usually take big decisions seriously, like marriage or changing jobs. Let us do everything of any importance with intent, especially eating. We can prevent and change many unwanted habits with this simple technique. I told patients that if they went off The Rules, they should do it purposefully and make it count. My choice would be cheesecake—nothing better. But I would do it with intent, with a plan for what happens next. The rare times it happens, I immediately go back to The Rules. More commonly, people lose focus, eat without intent, create bad habits, and rapidly regain the weight.

We Think We Are Experts

People learn quickly, but we sometimes think we're better than we are. This happens at work, playing sports, investing in stocks, and dieting. In any diet, including The Rules, you will lose weight if you're strict, and it can soon seem easy. Weight loss can be quick and dramatic in a low-carbohydrate or glycemic index-based diet. If you don't have much weight to lose, you can reach your goal in a few months or less. As I mentioned, I've done this myself many times only to regain weight.

When you reach your goal, you think you're an expert. How can the diet fail? How could I possibly gain it back? Remember that millionaires in the stock market often think the same thing before the crash. Overconfidence leads to small changes in our habits. The stock investor makes increasingly risky trades, the young driver texts while driving, and the dieter thinks they can have one snack or meal off the plan. It starts with a large fries at McDonald's, one Thin Mint Girl Scout cookie, or my nemesis of the early 2000s, the Sourdough Jack Burger at Jack in The Box. (Do not eat one; you will be addicted.) You tell yourself you know what you're doing and can have it just once. You can, for a while. But then you do it a few days a week, then every day. At one point, I had an iced latte and coffee cake at

Starbucks every morning and a Sourdough Jack Burger most afternoons on the way to pick up my son.

Every time I gained my weight back, it was because of overconfidence. I thought I was an expert and could safely make a few changes to my healthy diet. Weeks or months later, after gaining most or all the weight back, I would admit to myself that I was no expert and would go back to a strictly enforced diet plan. I would lose weight, and the cycle would repeat, often with the same temptation, the Sourdough Jack Burger.

We Think We Can Eat in Moderation

When we reach our goal with a diet, we rarely think hard about how to keep it off. I ask people what they'll do after they reach their goal. Often, they mention the diet's maintenance phase. Another standard answer is that they will "eat in moderation" or "eat sensibly." You've heard that many times. It works if you can do it. But if you could eat in moderation all the time, you would have done it and would not be overweight. This is like the sage advice of an investment expert—buy low and sell high. Expert advice, except how do you know when the stock is low or high? With food, my idea of moderation may not be the same as yours. Similarly, many patients tell me moderate drinking is a six-pack of beer at night. I don't have that same definition.

With eating, I have seen advice for dieting to keep calories under 2000 a day. That may work for some, but it can cause weight gain in others, depending on what you eat to get the 2000 calories. In addition, if you're not measuring and weighing food, you are likely eating more than you think. You might say that a moderate dinner is one serving of chicken breast and one serving of white rice. But if you don't measure it, your chicken breast may be one and a half servings and your rice three servings.

Despite the arguments of old-school dietitians, what you eat to reach 2000 calories matters. Eating 2000 calories of lean meat and vegetables is a good day, but the same calories eating pastries and pasta is not. We store fat more efficiently when we eat sugar and refined carbohydrates than when we eat meat and vegetables.

The biggest problem with the recommendation of eating in moderation is that even with the best intentions, it's difficult for most of us. Try to tell an alcoholic to drink alcohol in moderation. Can a drug addict do drugs in moderation? I'm the same way with bad carbs. One cookie leads to the next. My wife can eat one bite of cheesecake or a few M and M's. Watching her do it is annoying since I can't do it myself, at least not reliably. How many times do we tell ourselves, "Just one bite"? We know a moderate snack would be a handful of nuts or a few chips, but we keep going back. I call that eating from the trough, and I'll discuss how to avoid it later in the book. I'll give you a hint—it involves the analogy of alcohol again.

We Do Not Realize That Sugar and Carbohydrates Are Like an Addiction

Anyone reading this book has had a weight problem or knows someone who does. My weight is under control, but that has been far from the case for most of my life. Most of us will attest that it is hard to eat less sugar and refined carbohydrates, and it's hard to have one

Oreo cookie. Since we store fat efficiently when we eat sugar and carbohydrates, this is a genuine problem.

When I mention the low glycemic diets and The Three Rules, virtually all my patients do one of two things. They either say, "I love carbs." Or they think, "I love carbs." We developed a taste for carbohydrates over thousands or even millions of years. Lions like meat; we like carbohydrates. That is how our species has survived. With all the other wonderful traits of humans that have helped us—intelligence, opposable thumbs, and love for our family—we also developed a love of sweets. This has helped us survive—until recently.

Are sugar and refined carbohydrates addictive? Most overweight people believe they are. Some studies suggest it, and experts are divided on the issue. Again, I point to Gary Taubes's superb book, *The Case Against Sugar*, if you want to read about sugar addiction. But I don't care about science in this instance. Whether sugar and carbs are as addictive as cocaine doesn't matter to me. Sugar acts like an addictive substance. There are many definitions of addiction, but I consider something addictive if we do it despite the negative consequences, we try to stop and have trouble, we hide our behavior from others, or we are embarrassed by the behavior. I knew many years ago that sugar and carbs made me gain weight, and I remember hiding candy wrappers from my parents. I was embarrassed when I had to admit to my wife that I had a large fries at McDonald's when I bought our son a Happy Meal. I know this isn't the same as sneaking Johnny Walker at work, but it sounds like an addiction to me.

The point is not whether it is more difficult to quit sweets or drugs. But if you don't recognize that sugar and processed carbohydrates act like addictive substances, you will be tempted by a small treat. That's fine for some people, but not most of us; we don't stop at one. That leads to a rapid increase in the consumption of these foods. Then, most of the hard work is ruined, and you gain your weight back, usually quickly. The All or None approach works for other addictions, like alcohol and gambling. It works for sugar and refined carbohydrates. In the past, I have eaten all—now I eat none.

Part 2

Possible Solutions

Every diet works if you can stick to it.
That is the rub.

have already discussed some methods people use to lose weight. Countless books, magazines, websites, and videos are devoted to one diet or another. Every popular diet will cause weight loss; it won't be popular for long if it doesn't work. I've lost weight by cutting back, calorie counting, low-carbohydrate diets, and extreme exercise.

I lost weight faster in some diets than others, but they all worked when I stuck to them. That's the problem—all plans stop working if you stop following them. The key is finding a program you can stick to. You should learn about the options; some you can do on your own, and some involve a physician with supervised plans, medications, or surgery.

Most do-it-yourself plans are challenging, while physician-managed plans are often restrictive, expensive, and short-term, so regaining weight in both settings is typical. Medications for weight loss should not be taken forever, and most people gain weight back when they stop the drugs. Weight loss surgery works and has reasonably good long-term data supporting it. But it's drastic, forever changes how you eat, and has substantial risks.

In this chapter, I will review some of these methods for losing weight. They may be suitable for some people and may work for you. In my experience with weight problems and with my patients, there are too many failures with these plans for me to recommend them widely. I want a safe method that will work the first time and forever. The Three Rules is hard, but it is such a plan. If you follow it, you will still enjoy eating, lose weight, and not gain it back. You will also have the satisfaction that you did it on your own. That will help you in other aspects of your life. If you can lose weight on your own, what can't you do?

Eat Less

My doctor told me to stop having intimate dinners for four. Unless there were three other people.
Orson Welles

Historically, we dieted by eating less. Even before the word calorie was used, people knew that if you ate more, you would gain weight. If you ate less, you would lose weight or at least not gain. It isn't the weight of food that matters, but the calories, the amount of energy food has. A full plate of cabbage has fewer calories and less potential for weight gain than a small plate of cheesecake. Before we started eating so much sugar and carbohydrates, calories consumed and burned explained most weight gain and loss.

In general, eating less will result in weight loss. That is obvious. I have heard people, even health professionals, say that someone struggling with weight loss is not losing weight because they are not eating *enough*. That isn't true. Think about it. When a person eats nothing, they waste away and starve to death. If you feed them, they stop losing weight and eventually regain it. If zero food causes weight loss and starvation, how could it be that not eating enough would cause weight gain or interfere with weight loss?

Eating less helps with weight loss, but trying to fight appetite, our strongest urge, usually fails. Eating less is the basis of the diets I will discuss in this chapter. These diets work for many people, though usually only for a short time. You're welcome to try these diets—I have. If you want a plan that works, is easier than just eating less, and lasts forever, I would look elsewhere.

Just Cut Back

Can you cut back on what you eat and lose weight? The idea is simple. Eat less by cutting portion size, minimizing snacks, or eliminating certain fattening foods. I had a friend who could simply stop drinking alcohol for a few months and lose weight. When I asked patients if they were trying to do something about their weight, they often said they were cutting back on portion size. Sometimes, cutting back is effective, but usually, it takes more effort than that. Occasionally, a young, very active man cuts back and is successful. He stops eating desserts and second servings at meals. He may give up fast food or eating out entirely. The most successful will sometimes tell you that is all they have done, and they may even believe it. But if you delve deeper, you usually find they also gave up alcohol, sugary drinks, and refined carbohydrates. They may have started working out nearly every day. A lifestyle change that involves cutting back, giving up carbs, and exercising works, but only a few people do all that.

A few fortunate people can lose weight without much effort by cutting back and exercising a little more. I'm very happy for them. The problem is that they usually don't keep it up. They generally experience the yo-yo effect. They go on vacation and eat sweets again. They get busy at work and stop exercising. Stressful life situations lead to drinking alcohol. And so on. Then they gain the weight back and have to start over.

Far more common is that you try cutting back, not realizing how hard it is. (See the earlier chapter on the difficulty of losing weight.) You hear of a friend's success in cutting back, and you try it. You may not put in the effort that your friend did. Maybe you still have wine, don't exercise, and continue eating out too much. You fail and feel bad about yourself. Sometimes, we think there is something medically wrong with us, that our friend lost weight by cutting back and we cannot. But often, they were doing things we weren't doing; in any case, not everyone is the same. Some people can do certain things better than others, in weight loss and everything else.

Losing weight is hard. Cutting back on what you eat is relatively easy, but it rarely works. When it does, it isn't sustained, and you'll probably regain the weight quickly. If you are overeating, you should cut back but don't expect a significant improvement in your weight. There are better ways to lose weight in the long run.

Calorie Counting

What about formal calorie counting? You can have some success in counting and cutting calories, and it seems simple—eat fewer calories than you burn. Some smartphone apps allow you to scan the barcodes of products, search vast databases, and track calories, fat grams, carbohydrate content, and vitamins with no effort. Tracking calories isn't the problem.

The first issue is how low your calorie count must be to lose weight. Everyone is different. I'm about 5 foot 5 inches. Two thousand calories a day might cause a man 6 foot 5 to lose weight while I would gain weight. We also know that not all calories are the same. Eighteen hundred calories a day of protein, vegetables, and some fat would cause weight loss. Eighteen hundred calories of mashed potatoes and pie wouldn't. In addition, our energy expenditure affects the success of calorie counting. One hundred years ago, when people burned thousands of calories a day managing their home, they might have lost weight at 2200 calories. Today, with the tools we have for every chore in the house, you would probably gain weight at that calorie intake. That said, virtually everyone loses weight if they consume fewer than 1200 calories daily.

Most people who count calories eat more than they think. We talked of serving sizes earlier in this book. The standard serving size of boneless, skinless chicken breast is four ounces, but the average breast is six to seven ounces. I opened a Costco package, and one of the breasts was ten. A serving of pasta is two ounces, ⅛ of a box. If you are not measuring and weighing your food, you're likely underestimating what you're eating. With the analogy of alcohol, when I asked a patient how much they drank, if they said, "two drinks," and they were not measuring, they were probably drinking two rather large drinks, more than the standard five ounces of wine or one and a half ounces of spirits. So, when someone tells me they are not losing weight despite eating only 1100 calories a day, I first ask whether they weigh and measure their food. If not, then I know that they're undercounting. People also don't realize that if you're counting calories, every calorie matters. The small sample at Costco, the coffee creamer in the morning, the few fries from your son's dinner—it all counts. Twelve hundred calories isn't a lot. A few uncounted bites, each at forty calories, can make a difference.

Accurately counting calories is difficult enough, but being hungry is the hardest part. Remember, we have potent appetites that kick in *before* we lose significant weight. If that were not the case, we would only eat after we had already started losing weight. That would lead to starvation if the food we just decided not to eat happened to be the last food we would see for several days. I mentioned before that when I was calorie counting, I knew whether I had lost weight before I got on the scale in the morning. If I was hungry, I had lost weight. I dislike the idea of being hungry for weeks or months while I'm trying to work and enjoy my life. What if I want to eat out and already had 900 calories that day? That leaves only a few hundred calories for dinner at a restaurant. A salad is about all there is, and that's with a low-calorie dressing on the side.

Even if it works initially, the body adjusts to a low-calorie diet. If you eat 1200 calories daily, your body adapts nearly to that level after only a few months. Now, eating over 1200 calories might cause weight gain, and I don't think you want to count every calorie you eat for the rest of your life to avoid going over 1200. Most people eventually return to their original 1800-2000 calorie diet and regain weight. This is detailed in earlier chapters, and this problem derails most calorie-cutting diets over time.

Weight Watchers

Several commercial programs and systems for losing weight involve cutting back on how much you eat. Some talk of portion size, while others have you divide meals into different categories or eat only when you are hungry. You check in with advisers, who help keep you on task. Weight Watchers, the most popular system, assigns points based chiefly on calories. Some foods, such as fruits, vegetables, and pure proteins, do not count.

Many programs, including Weight Watchers, meld a typical calorie-cutting diet with a low carbohydrate or low glycemic index diet. There is much to like about these systems, especially that they hold you accountable with frequent check-ins with advisers. But you still have to count points or pay close attention to what you're eating. To do so accurately, you have to weigh and measure. That is difficult at restaurants and becomes tiresome at home. You still must eat in moderation, holding yourself to a small serving of something you like. A food choice may have ten points, but only if you measure it correctly and don't have seconds or thirds. A system may say only to eat when you're hungry, but we already know that. Again, if we could eat moderately, we wouldn't need a diet.

The biggest problem is what to do if you reach your goal. What next? When I asked patients this question, they usually said they would continue with the maintenance program or do the system on their own. Later, at the next yearly physical, most of those on Weight Watchers had lost some weight, but not as much as they had intended. Most stopped the diet because of cost, time factors, or lack of interest. Over the next year or two, the majority regained their weight. I have seen only a few patients have long-term success with Weight Watchers or similar plans.

Intermittent Fasting

I will briefly mention intermittent fasting. This diet has many forms, but they all work the same way. You pick times or days when you eat little to nothing. You eat as you wish in the other parts of the day or week. For example, you may only eat during an eight-hour period each day, fasting the rest. Or you might eat very little twice a week and moderately the other five days. This 5/2 ratio is the basis of one of the more popular intermittent fasting diets. The hope is that you cut enough calories while fasting to lose weight. Studies have been mixed, but most confirm that people can lose weight this way, and there may be additional health benefits unrelated to weight loss. It's easy and enjoyable for some, but most people don't reach their goal, and few keep the weight off. The diet may not work for most in the long run, but the benefits may be worth exploring if you're motivated.

In the actual world, things are different than in studies. People are often stricter with their diet when in a study, and being willing to participate requires a level of commitment we don't always see outside of a study protocol. There are at least three problems with intermittent fasting as it applies to weight loss. First is that some people overeat during the periods they are not fasting. If you are on the two-day/five-day intermittent fast, you may overeat enough during the five days to balance the two days when you eat little. You can become discouraged because you suffer during the fast and don't accomplish much.

Another problem is that the fasting periods can be challenging. Remember, if you could tolerate fasting and hunger, you likely wouldn't be overweight in the first place. This has been my problem when I've tried intermittent fasting. I am hungry and don't function very well when I'm hungry.

The most significant difficulty with this diet approach is social. What about travel? What if someone wants you to eat with them during a fast period, such as on vacation? What about long term? Do you want to be on such a regimen forever? My patients who did intermittent fasting would often return from vacation, no longer following the plan. They may have regained some weight and hoped to return to intermittent fasting, but it didn't happen. I never saw a patient stay on such a program long enough to lose all the weight they had planned. If I ever saw anyone lose weight and keep it off after one year, I do not recall it.

Jenny Craig, Nutrisystem, And Others

I have tried Jenny Craig, Nutrisystem, and similar programs and have lost weight every time. As most of you know from ads or trying them yourself, you eat the food they make. In some plans, you eat their food exclusively; in others, you supplement their food with healthy meals you prepare. The plans are regimented, so you have little opportunity to stray from what they tell you to do unless, of course, you eat food other than what they send you. When I tried such a diet, not being that picky, I was okay with the taste and quality of the food.

The meals and snacks are low-calorie, either because they are very healthy or small servings of less healthy food.

These programs are low-calorie diets, though some also have low carbohydrate and low glycemic options. The primary benefit is that they do nearly everything for you. You follow what they tell you. There are sometimes coaches and mentors, and that helps. I mentioned the flaw. It is still up to you not to stray from their plan. What if you want to go out to eat? What if you travel? What if you're hungry despite eating all your daily meals and snacks? If I have the willpower to eat only healthy foods in moderation, it isn't the actual preparation of the food that is the problem. I can look up a recipe, calculate the correct serving size, and make it myself. My challenge has always been eating in moderation, healthy or not, regardless of who prepares the food.

Like Weight Watchers, you also have the problem of what to do when you're done. Even if you stick it out for several months, eating only their food, and you lose the weight you hope to lose—then what? Are you going to eat their food forever? Some quit the program and make the foods they remember eating for the past few months. You will likely overeat if you're not careful and don't weigh and measure. If you can make sensible meals and not stray, why were you unsuccessful when you attempted that before? These diets can be more difficult in the long run than Weight Watchers because even if you are successful, you haven't learned how to lose weight and keep it off without the help of someone else making your meals. With The Three Rules, you learn how to lose weight, and you learn right away.

Follow The Rules, and you will succeed. That is all you need to know, forever.

Meal Replacement Diets

Jenny Craig and similar programs make meals for you, hoping you won't also eat extra food. Meal replacement plans are more restrictive. They give you food but not traditional meals—usually shakes, bars, and puddings. Years ago, at least twice, I lost weight on SlimFast. There are now a few different programs in SlimFast, and the shakes have changed, but the concept is that you drink their shakes, usually twice a day. When I did it, you were told to make a sensible dinner. Like all diets, SlimFast and similar programs work if you stick to them. The appeal of such a plan is that you don't have to think about what you eat for most of the day. You drink their shakes, which I enjoyed, and forget about other food. I could do it for a while, but I always slipped up. I overate when I went out for my "sensible dinner," on vacation, or after I got bored with the shakes.

Some such programs are more extreme than others, and some have medical supervision. You meet with nurses and doctors and use their meal-replacement products. Besides the supervision, which is supposedly tailored to your individual needs, there is little difference between doctor-supervised meal replacement diets and those you do on your own. The cost of the supervised plans is higher, and you usually can't buy their products online or at Target, as you can with SlimFast. They are low-calorie, generally less than a thousand per day, and the evidence shows that these diets work. But again, the long-term success rates are low for the same reasons the do-it-yourself programs usually fail. No one stays on them forever. I have nothing negative to say about supervised meal replacement programs. These programs are the same as almost all diets—they work when you do them and fail when you don't.

If you eat less, you will lose weight. It doesn't matter if you count calories on your own or join Weight Watchers or any other programs I mention. But the same problems arise in all of them. What have you learned from the diets? Do you want to be hungry forever or drink two or three shakes daily forever? What about travel, restaurants, and the simple boredom of eating their food? Most people regain a significant proportion of their lost weight soon after stopping the diets, even if a maintenance program is offered. The best way to lose weight and keep it off is to have a single plan that works forever. Sure, you have to stick to it, but The Three Rules will work better than these diets; it is essentially free and never stops working. Sticking to Three Rules is much easier than buying shakes or special meals for the rest of your life.

Exercise

Exercise will help you lose weight.
But to overcome a poor diet, it takes a lot of exercise.

Exercise burns energy. As we know, you will gain weight if you take in more fuel (calories) than you burn. We've discussed that certain foods may change how efficiently we gain weight, but the calorie concept is still generally true. So, doesn't it make sense that burning more energy will help with weight loss? Yes, of course, exercise helps with weight loss. But exercising enough to lose weight and keep it off is difficult. It can be done, and I know people who have done it. But it takes hard work, consistently, forever.

Should You Exercise?

It has been known for generations that exercise is good for us, and I cannot think of any medical condition harmed by exercise. Cardiovascular exercise, such as running or biking, and resistance training, such as weightlifting, help prevent disease. Exercise can lower the risk of heart disease, stroke, cancer, depression, erectile dysfunction, low back pain, and on and on. [14] [15] A recent extensive study

[14] Esposito K, Giugliano F, Di Palo C, et al. Effect of lifestyle changes on erectile dysfunction in obese men: a randomized controlled trial. JAMA. 2004;291(24):2978-2984. doi:10.1001/jama.291.24.2978

[15] Thorogood A, Mottillo S, Shimony A, et al. Isolated aerobic exercise and weight loss: a systematic review and meta-analysis of randomized controlled trials. Am J Med. 2011;124(8):747-755. doi:10.1016/j.amjmed.2011.02.037

confirmed what we already knew—moderate exercise saves lives.[16] I recommended exercise for nearly every patient.

The most significant benefits may be mental. Exercise gives us a feeling of accomplishment, making us happier and more likely to do other healthy things for ourselves. Exercise also relieves stress and anxiety. If I struggle to keep up with my wife when biking up a hill or with my son and nephew hiking in Montana, I am not worrying about other things in my life.

Nearly every healthy person benefits from exercise. When a patient saw me for an ailment, I usually recommended exercise as part of their recovery. Since exercise is challenging, most people exercise much less than recommended. The concept that exercise is good for us is well known, and I doubt I need to convince you. But will you lose weight if you exercise if you don't also change your diet?

Exercise And Weight Loss

Exercise helps people lose weight,[17] but less than you probably think. In multiple studies, exercise alone results in a loss of about 3 pounds and an inch of waist circumference. Many people fail to lose significant weight or even gain weight despite fairly rigorous exercise. If you look at charts that show calories burned with exercise or the

[16] Kraus WE, Powell KE, Haskell WL, et al. Physical Activity, All-Cause and Cardiovascular Mortality, and Cardiovascular Disease. Med Sci Sports Exerc. 2019;51(6):1270-1281. doi:10.1249/MSS.0000000000001939

[17] Thorogood A, Mottillo S, Shimony A, et al. Isolated aerobic exercise and weight loss: a systematic review and meta-analysis of randomized controlled trials. Am J Med. 2011;124(8):747-755. doi:10.1016/j.amjmed.2011.02.037

displays on the exercise machines, you can burn hundreds of calories in an hour. The machines overestimate the calories burned, but even at face value, that is not many calories. If you work out for 45 minutes and burn 300 calories, you can negate it with a Gatorade, a smoothie, or a snack. We eat far more food than our body needs, and burning 300 calories doesn't counteract our eating.

Remember that many years ago, the average person exercised far more than 45 minutes to get work done around the house. And that was while eating fewer carbohydrates and much less sugar. With the modern diet and our leisurely lives, this level of exercise won't cause dramatic weight loss. Most people do little or no hard exercise routinely. Many of my patients said they walked ten thousand steps as measured by a wrist monitor. Walking ten thousand steps during a regular day differs from an extra workout of ten thousand steps running or power walking. Before measuring, they may have been walking six thousand steps, so an additional four thousand around the office won't do much. If someone exercises for two hours or runs 10 miles every day, they will lose a lot of weight, but that isn't a reality for most of us.

I am not saying you shouldn't exercise. Everyone should. The benefits are enormous, and I will discuss them in more detail later in the book. I have never felt bad about myself after exercising and have never regretted working out. But I know that while exercise helps us lose weight and keep it off, it is nowhere near as important as what we eat.

Carbohydrate Based Diets

We all like sugar. That is a fact. It causes weight gain. That is another fact.

From what you have read in this book, you know I am against eating sugar, at least food with added sugar. There is no question that the quantities we consume can lead to obesity, diabetes, and many other illnesses. Cutting added sugar and certain other carbs out of your diet helps. I have already mentioned the Atkins Diet and the similar ketogenic diet, the prototype of very low-carb diets. These diets work, and I've said how they can fail in the long term. I want to expand on these diets because they are very tempting. I will also review the low glycemic index diets that arose from the low-carb diets. The ketogenic diet has made a comeback, and I will discuss it in more detail. The Three Rules is based on the glycemic index, but as you will see in later chapters, it's simpler and avoids the pitfalls of the diets I describe here.

Very Low-Carb Diets

Robert Atkins should be commended for popularizing the idea that cutting all sugar and nearly all carbs from the diet results in weight loss. The original Atkins Diet allowed for minimal carbohydrates, often fewer than 20 grams a day, less than what is in a single apple. Despite early and persistent condemnation by nutritionists and physicians, very low carbohydrate diets have been shown to work without being overly dangerous. As I related earlier, I lost 25 pounds in six weeks when I was on it. That is the rule, not the exception.

Like every diet and most things we do, these diets have some risks. Fortunately, most people do not have the dangerous rise in cholesterol predicted when the diets became popular. Every few years, researchers publish observational studies purported to show the cardiovascular risks of the diet, but these are not prospective and not convincing.

A high-protein, high-fat diet can lead to gout, a painful inflammation of one or more joints, constipation, and a few minor issues. Because the diet lacks fruit and vegetables, it is recommended to take a multivitamin. A rare person (and I was one) can develop dangerously high cholesterol levels, but overall, it's a reasonably safe way to lose weight, at least in the short term.

Over time, the Atkins Diet has been changed, now permitting a small amount of fruit and vegetables. Once you have progressed on the diet, you can slowly start eating other foods with carbs, again only in small amounts. The currently popular ketogenic diet is like the original Atkins Diet, stressing fat more than protein, but we can think of it as the same as the Atkins diet.

People often misuse the term keto and think they are on a keto diet when they are just eating fewer carbs than before. The media and many researchers studying low-carb diets make the same mistake; they use 25% of daily intake as the threshold for a low-carb diet. Headlines will read, "Ketogenic diet is no more effective than cutting calories," or "Ketogenic diet causes heart attacks." If the study relies on reports from participants, they are probably eating more than 25%. That is not a ketogenic or Atkins diet. The original Atkins Diet allowed 20-30 grams of carbs daily, which converts to 80-120 calories from carbs. That's about 5% of a daily calorie intake.

Products labeled "keto" or "keto-friendly" have no standard meaning, and most haven't been studied to see what happens to your metabolism. Ketogenesis is when animals break down fat and sometimes protein to make ketones, an alternative fuel to glucose. This occurs in times of starvation and when carbohydrate intake is very low. Historically, this diet was used to treat childhood epilepsy and a few other conditions. Dr. Atkins recognized that it would also cause weight loss and recommended testing the urine for ketones to ensure that ketosis was maintained.

A true ketogenic diet requires you to make ketones. To do so, most people must limit their carb intake to about 20 grams a day. If you're not paying close attention and counting everything, you will quickly eat more than that. As mentioned above, one apple is about 20 grams. Patients tell me they are "doing keto" but are eating fruit, vegetables, and whole-grain bread. They may be on a healthy diet and may even lose weight, but they are not on a ketogenic diet. This haphazard approach usually fails over time. More bad carbs creep into their diet, and weight loss ceases. Worse, they will gain weight if they eat these foods and think that allows them to overindulge in sweets later in the day.

I sometimes recommend the ketogenic diet for patients discouraged by other diets, especially if they have significant weight to lose. The actual ketogenic diet is reliable and fast. If you stick to it, you can lose 20 pounds in the first month. But I don't like these diets for the long term. First, there is no reason to be that restrictive. You can lose weight, though maybe not as quickly, if you eat fruits, vegetables, beans, and nuts. I typically eat over 150 grams of carbs daily, but I don't eat bad carbs. This is healthier than keto since these foods have health benefits in addition to being compatible with weight loss. While not as harmful as once thought, eating meat, especially processed red meat, and eggs in sizable amounts indefinitely isn't a great idea. Cheese, which has been shown to be safe and perhaps beneficial, has not been studied long term in the massive quantities some people on the Atkins and keto diets consume. But even if you wanted to eat that way forever, almost no one does. They tire of eating with such little variety, and if you stick it out and lose all the weight you plan to lose, then what? As with the other plans I mentioned, you haven't learned anything and will probably return to what you did before. You might try to moderate your carb intake, but you know how difficult it is to moderate.

Soon, I will teach you how The Rules work. Some products labeled "keto" or "keto-friendly" are acceptable, depending on the ingredients. But you must be careful. A keto brownie might have a few grams of added sugar. What if you ate six brownies in a day, plus other carbs? I doubt you would be burning fat and making ketones. A square of a Hershey bar has under 2 grams of carbs, making it "keto-friendly." Great. But I can't stop at one square. A ketogenic diet means that you are always or nearly always in a state of ketogenesis.

That requires constant attention to how much you're eating. I find that difficult and not much different than counting calories.

Since The Three Rules is the best solution, I didn't talk much to patients about low-carb diets. But when I did, I recommended they start the ketogenic diet and quickly move to The Three Rules. They could gain confidence from the rapid weight loss and see how harmful sugar is. Once following The Three Rules, they learned to eat a healthy diet, lose weight, and keep it off forever.

Low Glycemic Diets

Soon after it became apparent that the Atkins Diet and similar low-carb diets caused weight loss, many related diets were created. Most of these were lumped together as "modified Atkins Diets," and you will still hear the term. In my experience, The South Beach Diet, developed by Arthur Agatston, MD, is the most important of them. I followed this diet off and on for many years and found it less restrictive and more enjoyable than the Atkins Diet. I lost weight, perhaps not as fast as with Atkins, but fast enough, and I kept the weight off—when I stuck to it.

All the diets in this category look at the glycemic index and, to a lesser extent, the glycemic load. As you recall, the glycemic index refers to how much your blood glucose rises after eating something that contains 50 grams of carbohydrates. Foods with added sugar and processed, refined carbohydrates score higher on the glycemic index. Proteins and fats are zero, having little or no effect on glucose in the blood, and most fruits and vegetables are low. Glycemic load considers how much you eat at a time, roughly equivalent to a serving size on the package. (We all know we usually eat more than the serving size listed.)

We gain weight when we eat enough high-glycemic foods. The worst foods have both a high glycemic index and glycemic load. These foods, such as potatoes, are densely packed with carbs, so one serving gives you a significant amount, often more than 50 grams. And gram for gram, those carbs raise your sugar significantly. When we avoid high-glycemic foods, we lose weight.

The South Beach Diet and similar diet books explain the glycemic index and guide you to the foods that are okay to eat. But they can be complex to follow. I haven't read all of them, but The South Beach Diet allows some foods in the later phases of the diet that are not allowed early on. There are charts and tables explaining what you can eat and when, and you can do an internet search to find where a particular food falls on the diet. Most people I know, myself included, want to avoid memorizing tables or carrying notes when grocery shopping or eating out.

These diets also allow certain foods in small quantities. For example, during phase two of the South Beach Diet, you can have a serving of bread. That sounds like eating in moderation. If I could eat in moderation or stop after eating one dinner roll every time, I would never have had a weight problem. Allowing small amounts of certain foods at different times of the diet sounds excellent—more variety, more of what we like. But it also allows us to play mind games with ourselves. "I can have one roll. That was a small roll; I'll have half of another." Then, before you know it, you've had four.

The low glycemic diets work, and in a sense, The Three Rules is a low glycemic diet. But The Rules avoids the pitfalls of the South Beach and similar diets. It's better to have a few rules, even if they prohibit food categories entirely, than to allow some foods in moderation or require a complex system to remember. Using the analogy of alcohol again, it's like allowing an alcoholic a single 12-ounce bottle of light beer three times a week. It may seem harsher to prohibit all alcohol, but it works. Yes, the Three Rules prohibits foods with added sugar. But if you cut out most but not all food with added sugar, you will be frustrated and probably unsuccessful in your goal of weight loss and keeping it off. Nothing bothered me more in my days of dieting than giving up most of what I liked yet still not losing weight.

Medications and Surgery

When you cannot do something on your own, it is wise to ask for help.

Most overweight people have tried to lose weight, and many have had some success. Despite extreme effort, some people still cannot lose weight and ask their doctors for help; patients regularly asked me for medications or other interventions such as surgery. There is a stigma attached to drugs and surgery, but there shouldn't be. Why is obesity treatment somehow wrong, yet medication for cholesterol or surgery for a hernia is not? Many medical conditions cannot be treated without medicine or surgery.

That said, it's preferable to deal with weight on your own, if possible. You achieve a sense of accomplishment that leads to more lasting success, and you avoid the risks inherent to all medications and all surgery. You also save money, though that's a minor issue, since losing weight by any method, even surgery, saves money in the long run. I didn't prescribe medications or refer for surgery often, but I understand the benefits in some cases. I hope you try the Three Rules rather than go immediately to medical interventions, but it's worth knowing what else is available for people with a weight problem.

Weight-Loss Medications

The medications on the market today have benefits and are generally safe. Most are indicated for short-term use, but a few can be taken long-term. Physicians differ in their use of these medications and how often, and I only occasionally prescribed them.

Until recently, you could expect a 5% weight loss from a medication. That means if you weigh two hundred pounds and are obese, you will lose ten pounds in 6-12 months. That's fine, but with adherence to a diet such as The Three Rules, a 200-pound person who is 50 pounds overweight could lose 25-30 pounds or more in that time frame. In the last few years, a new group of weight-loss medications, the glucagon-like peptide-1 or GLP-1 agonists, was approved for weight loss. These medications act like the hormone GLP-1, which affects glucose control, appetite, and body weight. Initially developed to treat diabetes, they were quickly found to have a weight loss effect, as much as 10-15% of body weight.[18] They cause weight loss by multiple mechanisms, but one involves its potential side effects— nausea, loss of appetite, and other gastrointestinal symptoms.

Despite the sometimes impressive weight loss, I didn't recommend GLP-1 agonists for most people. There are always risks to medications, especially new ones, and in the study I reference, ten percent of people taking semaglutide (Wegovy and Ozempic) experienced severe adverse reactions. A new study released in

---

[18] Wilding JPH, Batterham RL, Calanna S, et al. Once-Weekly Semaglutide in Adults with Overweight or Obesity. N Engl J Med. 2021;384(11):989-1002. doi:10.1056/NEJMoa2032183

October 2023 showed an increased risk of pancreatitis, bowel obstruction, and gastroparesis (paralysis of the stomach).[19] Another concern I have with the GLP-1 medications is the loss of lean body mass. About 40% of the weight lost in those taking semaglutide was muscle. Frailty, a consequence of declining muscle mass, is a significant cause of morbidity and mortality as we age. It will be many years before we know the long-term risks of this class of medication. The financial cost is also a problem. Insurance plans usually don't cover weight loss drugs; when they do, there is often a significant copay. The drug cost is far more than that of a gym membership or any new foods you would buy with a healthier diet.

I didn't like giving weight loss medications for the same reason I don't like meal replacement plans. You haven't learned anything while taking weight loss drugs. When you go off a medication or fad diet, you will likely return to your previous eating habits because you didn't intentionally change much about your eating when you were on the medication or particular diet regimen. Do you want to take a medication forever to preserve a 20-pound weight loss? Staying on a diet with a few rules is better than taking medication forever. When stopping Ozempic and the other GLP-1 medications, you can expect to regain much of your lost weight.[20]

-----

[19] Sodhi M, Rezaeianzadeh R, Kezouh A, Etminan M. Risk of Gastrointestinal Adverse Events Associated With Glucagon-Like Peptide-1 Receptor Agonists for Weight Loss [published online ahead of print, 2023 Oct 5]. JAMA. 2023;10.1001/jama.2023.19574. doi:10.1001/jama.2023.19574

[20] Wilding, John P H, et al. (2022). Wilding JPH, Batterham RL, Davies M, et al. Weight regain and cardiometabolic effects after withdrawal of semaglutide: The STEP 1 trial extension. Diabetes Obes Metab. 2022;24(8):1553-1564. doi:10.1111/dom.14725

If you start by changing your eating habits with The Three Rules, you avoid medications, learn something, and lose weight. If you stick to the new lifestyle, you will keep the weight off.

Bariatric Surgery

Bariatric surgery refers to the surgical techniques designed to produce significant, sustained weight loss. I won't get into the details of the surgeries or make specific recommendations about when to consider bariatric surgery. I will discuss the benefits and risks of bariatric surgery in general.

After bariatric surgery, people lose weight, a lot of weight. Studies show that obese people often lose one hundred pounds or more with the most effective surgical techniques. As a percentage of total weight, 25% weight loss is common. You probably have seen people who have lost more than that. Surgery can reverse diabetes, sleep apnea, hypertension, and other conditions. Overall survival and quality of life both improve in most studies. Over time, some weight is regained, but not usually all of it.

So, what are the downsides? Surgery has risks, with the overall risks varying by surgery type. There is a risk of death from bariatric surgery, with most studies showing the 30-day mortality being between 0.2% and 0.5%. The overall complication rate is higher, but most surgical complications are successfully managed. Don't forget, though, that there is a significant mortality and morbidity risk from remaining obese. The life expectancy of the obese who don't lose weight is much lower than those who do.

Comparing the benefits and risks of obesity surgery is complex. Those who lose weight on their own, as you will if you follow The Three Rules, do so with negligible risk. Without a good plan, though, most people are unsuccessful on their own. There is another concept regarding the surgical risk that needs to be considered. Let's say a study shows that surgery has a 1% mortality risk at 30 days, but the risk of dying without surgery is 2% at ten years. (These are not the actual numbers with bariatric surgery, but the numbers are close enough for this example to help.) The 1% risk is right up front. If you are in that 1%, that's it; you are gone. If you don't have surgery and are in the 2% group who dies in the next ten years, you are likely to live several years. So, the overall death risk is higher without surgery in this example, but you may have a better overall likelihood of living several years.

Aside from surgical risks, a significant downside of bariatric surgery is that it will change your eating. Of course, that is part of the upside, but you will be completely unable to eat certain foods. You may get diarrhea, bloating, or vomiting if you eat foods you have loved for years. You may be at risk for anemia and vitamin deficiencies, and certain medications must be avoided. Lastly, many regain significant weight by finding ways to get calories and carbs.

All that said, there are excellent reasons to have bariatric surgery. If your doctor thinks you should have surgery, talk it over with them carefully and consider it. But, if you have not yet put all your effort into losing weight without surgery, I recommend trying that first. In the next section, you will learn why The Three Rules is the best solution to your weight problem.

Part 3

The Three Rules— The Best Solution

Why should others believe the promises I make to them if I don't keep the promises I make to myself?

Rules can have a negative connotation, and we often resent rules imposed by our parents, teachers, and bosses. Yet, to keep some level of order, we need rules; having rules and principles to live by is helpful. The Three Rules to Lose Weight and Keep It Off Forever is a set of rules for eating that we impose on ourselves. If you don't like the word "rules," call them "promises to yourself."

The critical concept is eating with intent. Eating and drinking are perhaps the most essential actions of any animal's daily life, including ours. In today's world, nourishment is so plentiful that we don't think about it. Unlike other animals, we need to eat with intent, meaning we must think about what we eat. Animals in the wild don't, and humans before us didn't have this luxury. To survive, we had to eat everything we encountered that wasn't toxic; now, rarely truly hungry, we should think about everything we eat. Do I want to eat from a bowl of candy? Do I need to keep Doritos in the house and eat them whenever I want? Should I eat the apple in the fridge? It's a valuable concept for everything we do. Do everything, including eating, with intent.

We have discussed some key points of the diet, and I will now go over the actual Rules. I will show you that while The Rules require effort, you will live a normal, happy life. Losing weight and keeping it off, the goal of The Three Rules, will give you improved health, help prevent disease, improve your quality of life, and allow you to be more active and participate in more rewarding activities as you age.

The Rules will change how you eat, but you will still enjoy eating. You will be satisfied, have many food options, and be able to travel and eat at restaurants with little difficulty. I wrote this section of the first edition right after Thanksgiving. I had turkey, ham, Brussels sprouts, green beans, beet hummus with vegetables (very good; my niece made it), Greek salad, and assorted cheeses. I didn't eat the pumpkin cheesecake or mashed potatoes. It was a good Thanksgiving with my family, and I didn't feel deprived. I was also one of the few who didn't complain of feeling tired and bloated afterward. Last year, we went out to dinner for Thanksgiving (the first time) at my favorite seafood restaurant. I had a crab cocktail, sautéed scallops, roasted mushrooms, and green beans. No dessert. I had nothing to regret the following morning. Since I don't drink alcohol (though, as you will see, it isn't prohibited in The Rules), I didn't have a glass of wine either.

The Rules are all about what to remove from your diet. There isn't a single food that causes weight loss. On the web, there are ads for "fat-burning foods" or "cardiologist says this food will cause weight loss." Not true. All diets work by removing something from what you usually eat—calories, carbs, sugars, fats, whatever. The Three Rules involves removing what I call **bad carbs** from your diet. Another term I will use for "bad carbs" is **junk food**. There are various definitions of junk food, but when I use it, I mean bad carbs.

There are three categories of **bad carbs**; in The Three Rules, you remove all of them. When you do that, you have to eat something. So, you eat good carbs, proteins, and fats. These good foods are not the cause of the weight loss. They are what you eat after removing the fattening foods. A steak does not cause weight loss, but it allows for the weight loss that occurs after removing the four donuts from your diet.

You have heard The Rules earlier in the book to some extent, but we must be clear on exactly what The Rules means. The Rules are simple, but they are strict. Those who haphazardly follow The Rules sometimes succeed but usually do not. Following any diet only partially can lead to giving up some of what you like and failing in your ultimate weight loss goal. This causes frustration, and you will probably quit the diet. If you are strict, The Rules work.

The Three Rules are not perfect. It would be nice if every food group could be absolutely good or bad. That is not how nature behaves. Fortunately, there are only a few foods in this gray area. I avoid these. Why risk it? There are so many other choices. Two examples of gray area foods are ripe bananas and brown rice. Neither one fits perfectly into a Rule. I don't eat either. Both are easily avoided. Why ruin a diet with a few avoidable foods?

Dieters find it challenging to accept that the "All or None" approach works best. When starting The Three Rules, it seems hard to believe I am asking you to give up bread, sugar, potatoes, or something else altogether, 100%. It may be difficult in the plan's first few days or weeks. You are used to eating a piece of candy in the afternoon or a roll with dinner. But giving it up completely is far easier than having a little. I repeat it over and over because it's true. You would never recommend that a reformed alcoholic have a small beer after work or treat themselves to a shot of tequila on a holiday. One drink will not hurt them, but they can't stop at one drink. A cookie won't hurt me, but I can't stop at one cookie. It's the same thing. I don't believe in cheat days or treats. An occasional treat becomes a daily one, which is the same as a habit.

All or None is the scariest part of the Three Rules and its greatest strength. Committing to it is daunting, but you will succeed. If a person with an addiction commits to conquering alcohol or drugs, they give them up completely. If they do that, they are sure to succeed. If you completely give up the bad carbs outlawed by the Three Rules, your success is nearly inevitable.

I will review each Rule and common issues people have when implementing it. The Rules sound straightforward, and they are. But foods are not always simple in themselves, and we eat foods with many components. Foods are marketed to sound healthy, and food labels don't always tell the complete picture.

I hope you will agree that The Rules are more straightforward than guidelines, charts, counting, and measuring; carbs are easier to control than hunger; giving up some groups of foods is more manageable than cutting back on all food. In the later sections, you will learn a few issues specific to keeping weight off forever. I will help with some tricks, pointers, and pitfalls and discuss other aspects of eating and lifestyle that might apply. You will realize that, as with anything, even an excellent plan has downsides. If you follow The Three Rules, the benefits greatly outweigh the negatives.

As with anything we do, The Three Rules has risks. For most people, the risks are very low. Discussing this or any significant change in your diet with your doctor is always a good idea.

Rule One:
Do Not Eat Food with Added Sugar

Sugar has been called the new smoking.
I don't know if it's that bad, but it's bad.

I have discussed why sugar causes weight gain. When we eat sugar, our blood glucose rises, triggering the rise in fat-storing hormones, especially insulin. The degree to which specific foods raise sugar is testable and described by the terms glycemic index and glycemic load. Added sugar raises our blood glucose the most, and the more you eat, the worse it is. But as you know, moderation and limiting yourself to a little of something is very difficult.

General Concepts and Common Foods

There is sugar in fruit, vegetables, beans, nuts, and dairy. This has no bearing on Rule 1. We are talking about sugar added to the otherwise healthy good carbs, protein, and fat in your food. I will say it many times, but here it is. Sugar put into a food product or a dish you make at home will rapidly raise your blood glucose and make it easy to gain weight and difficult to lose it. Don't eat it if sugar is added. Read the ingredients section of the food label. You can look at the Nutrition Facts section and see that there may be grams of sugar in foods like mixed nuts, but if no sugar is added, you can eat it (unless it breaks another Rule).

Most of the foods off limits because of Rule 1 are obvious. At a store, foods are packaged and processed, and they report the sugar on the label. But you have to look carefully. Sugar has many names: corn syrup, evaporated cane juice, rice syrup, dextrose, sucrose, glucose, fruit juice concentrate, honey, maltodextrin (not quite sugar, but close enough), molasses, and many more. I was tempted to list all the ones I could find, but it became ridiculous. Instead, I have referenced the University of California website in the footnote for more details.[21] Some types of sugar may be a little better than others, but for me, an All or None eater, it only works if you avoid all of it. When in doubt regarding an ingredient, look it up.

Be wary of seemingly healthy foods like granola. Most granola is a mixture of nuts, processed oats (against Rule 2), and a sugar-sweetener, sometimes honey. Honey is just dissolved sugar made by bees rather than humans. I don't know how granola ever became considered healthy. It may have a few benefits, but it definitely will raise your blood sugar. Trail mix is another example. There is often granola, sugar-sweetened fruit, and sometimes even candy. Just because someone says a food is healthy doesn't mean it won't make you fat.

If you are making the food at home, it's easier to know what is off-limits since you add the sugar yourself—think of how much sugar you add to cookies, pastries, sweetened sauces, and candy. But you

---

[21] https://sugarscience.ucsf.edu/hidden-in-plain-sight/#.XeJajJNKi8U

must also consider some sweeteners that don't sound like sugar. Adding corn syrup to your Christmas cookies is the same as adding sugar.

It is more challenging to follow Rule 1 when someone else makes your food, and you don't see the labels, such as in restaurants. Some restaurants list ingredients—not quite as trustworthy as a packaged product's label, but it's pretty good. Most of the hidden sugar in restaurants is in the sauces and dressings. Don't be afraid to ask the wait staff if sugar is added. If they are unsure, or you don't trust the answer, skip the sauce or tell them to put it on the side. Usually, a quick taste will tell you if significant sugar is added, but not always. If you want to be strict, get a dish that is definitely free of added sugars: most meat, chicken, and fish dishes can be made with no sweetened sauces. For salads, bleu cheese, a simple vinaigrette, and oil and vinegar are usually safe.

- Read every label's ingredient list.
- Confirm there is no added sugar.
- Double-check that there is no added sugar by a different name.

Can I Eat Any Sugar?

Once you know the Rule, there is nothing to understanding it. Do not eat food with added sugar. But that doesn't mean that you don't eat any sugar. Because sugar is a component of so many foods, people get it wrong all the time. When I tell people this Rule, they ask, "You don't eat any sugar?" I do eat sugar. I eat the sugar in most natural foods—fruit, vegetables, beans, nuts, and dairy. Just because a food is natural doesn't mean it's healthy or suitable for this or any diet, but the sugars in most natural foods (other than honey) are fine. Almost all fruits have sugar, and nearly all fruits are acceptable on this diet. I eat at least three servings of fruit daily—apples, oranges, grapefruit, berries, whatever. Most of these fruits are sweet—not as sweet as candy—but sweet enough. And, if you don't eat sugar-sweetened foods, everything else tastes sweeter than it did before.

The key to this Rule is to read the label of every food you eat. Pay little attention to the grams of sugar in the "Nutrition Facts." If apples had labels, they would list about 20 grams of sugar. This is not added sugar. Some labels list added sugar grams, which is helpful; for The Three Rules, it should be zero. (A bottle of Mountain Dew has 77 grams of added sugar, the same as 19 white packets.) What difference does it make if the sugar is added or in the food naturally? Again, it comes down to glycemic index, how much your blood glucose rises after eating. The primary sugar in most fruit is fructose. At the levels in fruit, combined with the fiber in the fruit, your blood sugar doesn't rise much, and you cannot efficiently store fat. High fructose corn syrup is different; since it has so much fructose and glucose, it overwhelms your body. Your glucose level rises fast, allowing you to store fat efficiently. I will not even get into the other harmful effects of this food additive.

Many foods have no added sugar, yet there are grams of sugar listed on the label. These are all fine: milk, yogurt, nuts, vegetables, beans, most canned tomatoes, some tomato sauces, salad dressings (read the label carefully), and many more. A perfect example is the wonderful Costco plain nonfat Greek yogurt, with seven grams of carbohydrates and four grams of sugar per serving. Look at the label; in the ingredients, there is only milk. There is no sugar *added*. In the left column, you see 4 grams of sugar. That is all lactose. You can (and should) eat this on The Three Rules plan. I eat it with frozen berries for breakfast nearly every day. You put the yogurt and berries in a food storage container the night before, and it's perfect by morning. I sometimes add cinnamon or cocoa powder for a unique taste. While the fruit has fructose and the yogurt has lactose, neither raises blood glucose or fat-storing hormones much. Lately, I've been making Greek yogurt, and while the exact calories and carb content may be slightly different from Costco's, I certainly don't add sugar to mine. Make sure to read the labels. Most major yogurt brands have no added sugar, but some do, and some have ingredients against Rule 3. There is no reason to ruin a diet with Greek yogurt.

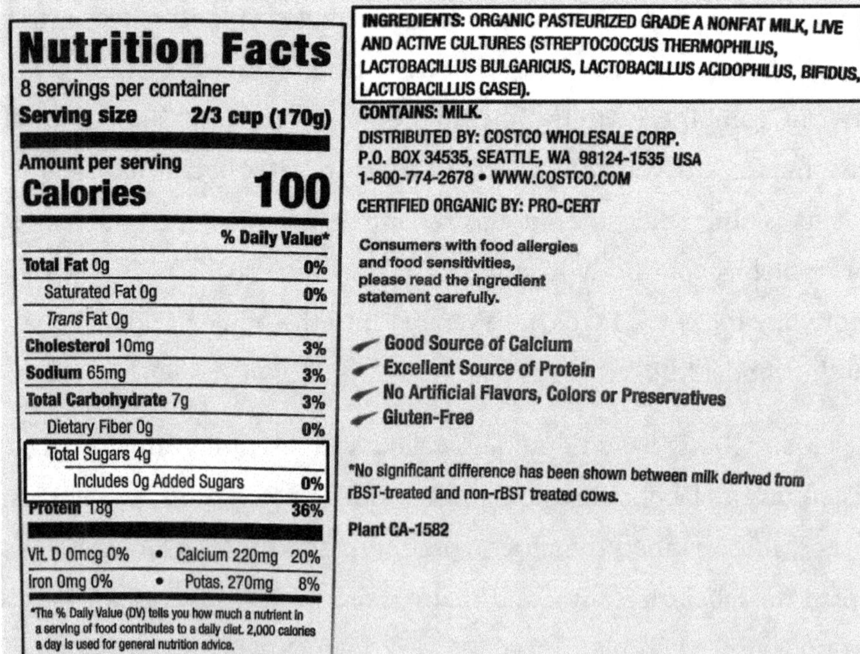

So, you can eat the sugars in most fruits, vegetables, beans, and nuts. Some fruits and vegetables are against Rule 3, but not many. Beans and nuts have almost no effect on blood glucose because of their fiber content and the types of sugar and starch they contain. If you stick to The Rules, even high-calorie nuts will allow for weight loss.

- Sugar in all its forms should not be in the ingredients.
- Grams of sugar in the Nutrition Facts do not matter as long as there is no added sugar.

If It's Not Sweet, Can I Eat It?

You might be surprised by some foods that have added sugar. Diced tomatoes, canned beans, and other canned vegetables sometimes have sugar in the ingredients. Again, most vegetables and all beans have grams of sugar in the nutrition facts, but the fiber prevents your glucose from rising quickly in your blood. Make sure there is no added sugar in the cans you buy. Even savory sauces can have sugar added. A few years ago, a patient told me he wasn't succeeding on the diet. He ate a lot of tomato sauce, and I asked him if sugar had been added. He said he didn't know. He had given up so many foods but hadn't lost weight. That was frustrating for him, but he wasn't reading the labels. I don't know if sugar was added to his sauce, but he may have been eating a lot of added sugar if he wasn't reading the labels. Condiments are also common sources of hidden sugar. Ketchup has about 3 grams of added sugar per tablespoon. Most people use far more than one tablespoon of ketchup, so that sugar adds up.

Many snack foods that are not sweet break Rule 1. Graham crackers are sweet enough to know that they are against the Rule. Would you think Rold Gold pretzels have added sugar? Read the label—corn syrup! There is just no way to know without reading the label. (Pretzels are also against Rule 2 because of the refined wheat in them.)

Protein bars are notorious. Both Clif Bars and Snickers bars have over 20 grams of added sugar. That isn't counting the other bad carbs in them. Granola bars can be just as bad. There are some low-sugar bars, but very few have zero sugar added. Don't assume that if a bar is labeled "low sugar," you can eat it. Low is not zero. Would five grams of added sugar in a protein bar derail your diet? Almost certainly not. But 5 grams several times a day will. Eating low-sugar foods in small amounts involves eating in moderation. As I repeatedly say, most of us cannot eat in moderation. I am best off choosing a snack with zero added sugar. Then I don't think about it. I snack on nuts, fruit, beef jerky (some jerky has sugar added), cheese, and many other foods. I don't find it difficult to survive. Another problem is that store-bought snacks usually have refined carbohydrates, breaking Rule 2.

- Most snack foods and protein bars have added sugar.
- Many sauces, even the savory ones, have added sugar.

Final Points on Rule 1

Rule 1 simply means giving up foods with added sugar. That isn't hard to follow in the long run, but it can be challenging when you start. It was a change for me to pay attention to sugar and to read every label. But once you get into the habit, it's easy; we tend to eat the same foods repeatedly. Most products are obvious, and you don't need to read the labels: candy, doughnuts, cookies—obviously out. For other things, I don't have to read many labels anymore since I stay with the same brands for my staple foods. I read the label for any new product I eat. A product similar to one I usually eat may have unexpected added sugar, but it may also have something against Rule 2 or 3. Don't forget that there are two more Rules, and all three must be observed.

Since the first edition was published, I've come across products that break Rule 1 with a negligible amount of sugar. The label lists dextrose or other sugars, but the Nutrition Facts section will say there are zero grams of sugar. The FDA (Food and Drug Administration) allows products with 0.5 grams of sugar and just under five calories per serving to be labeled zero sugar and sugar-free. A patient pointed out to me that iodized salt contains dextrose. I changed to sea salt for a while because dextrose isn't listed on the label. I learned that an entire container of table salt has less than one gram of dextrose. (Dextrose is necessary to stabilize the iodine.) One gram in a pound of salt is nothing, and I'm back to the inexpensive table salt. There are several products like this, including deli meats. If I go on a long drive and stop at a gas station, I sometimes eat packaged turkey. I will always try to find one with no sugar in the ingredients. But if my only food option in the store lists sugar but no carbohydrates or added sugars in the Nutrition Facts, I will eat it. At your home grocery store, there will be a better option.

Non-nutritive sweeteners (artificial and natural low-calorie sweeteners) can be problematic. Later, we'll talk about the potential risks of these products and which might be best. For now, I want you to know that some packets have substantial sugar, and I avoid packets of Splenda, Equal, and their generics, aspartame and sucralose for this reason. These contain about a half-gram of dextrose or maltodextrin per serving. One packet in a coffee shop is okay, but if you have cups of tea and coffee all day long, it adds up. The green stevia packets contain erythritol, a sugar alcohol, but no sugar. They don't affect The Three Rules but may have an additional risk we'll discuss.

I recommend avoiding anything that lists sugar in the ingredients. Still, if it's unavoidable, like deli meat with less than a gram, or table salt, where I confirmed the sugar content is negligible, you can eat it. I am not talking about addictive foods with a few grams of sugar per serving, bars with "low sugar on the label and bad carbs in the ingredient list, or any of the other dangers mentioned above.

Rule Two:
Do Not Eat Food with Processed and Refined Carbohydrates

Processing and refining may be good in some settings, but not when it comes to eating.

This Rule is more difficult to explain and more challenging to follow than Rule 1. I even had some difficulty coming up with the wording. First, I used only "processed," but that seemed to imply that even processing fruit into dried fruit, peanuts into peanut butter, or milk into yogurt somehow raised the glycemic index and made them against The Rules. I also tried "refined," but that was somewhat vague, and refining sounds like a good thing. Now, I use both words, knowing it isn't a simple rule to understand without further explanation. Processing means that something was done to the natural food before we eat it. When I use the word "refine," I mean that something good was changed or removed from the food. Note that none of this applies to foods such as meats and fats since they have no carbohydrates. Any form of meat or oil is fine.

The problem with processed, refined carbs is that they raise your blood glucose quickly, reflected in the glycemic index. Most unprocessed, natural foods like nuts, beans, fruit, vegetables, and some whole grains won't raise blood sugar high enough to interfere with weight loss. Processed and refined foods like flour and white rice will. The biggest culprits in this category are processed wheat products—bread, pasta, crackers, other snack foods, pastries, cookies, and breakfast cereal. The glycemic index skyrockets when the bran and fiber are removed from wheat. (This has nothing to do with gluten, which adversely affects some people, but is a protein and irrelevant to the Rules.) Most of these products also have added sugar and are against two of the Three Rules.

Not all processed foods are off-limits. Foods without carbs, such as processed meats, are acceptable in The Three Rules Plan. (There may be other health issues, but that is a topic for another book.) Even some processed foods with carbohydrates are acceptable in The Three Rules. Taking fruit, vegetables, nuts, and beans and chopping or mashing them doesn't significantly change the glycemic index, even though they are processed in one sense. Chopping and mashing fruit is fine, but removing fiber and pulp leaves only the sugars and raises the glycemic index. A popular dish now is mashed cauliflower. This is the same for your body as eating whole cauliflower. (Your stomach mashes in much the same way.) Peanut and other nut butters are just mashed nuts, and since nuts are good, then nut butter is also good. You must read the label because many nut butters and mashed fruit products have added sugars or other ingredients you want to avoid.

This brings us to one of the "gray area" foods I mentioned. My wife has pointed out to me many times over the years that not everything is black and white. I know that, but my brain has trouble accepting it. I told you that the Three Rules isn't perfect—nothing is. Richard Carlson taught that we should "make peace with imperfection," and I'm working on it. I have accepted that grains are in this category. If you eat unprocessed whole grains other than rice (we'll talk about rice later), the glycemic index is low, and you can eat it. I eat unprocessed barley several days a week. But if you grind it up fine enough, as in flour, then even if unrefined, your body digests and absorbs the carbs rapidly, your glucose rises, and you can gain weight. In other words, the glycemic index increases when you make flour from grain, even if you don't remove the bran. We'll discuss whole grains in the next chapter and again with Rule 3. **For now, know that all flour made from grain is against Rule 2.**

Most people find that Rule 2 is the hardest of The Rules to follow when they start. We don't go into withdrawals when we stop eating these foods, but we have habits of eating bread, cereal, pasta, and other refined-wheat products, and making these foods is easy and quick. Many of my patients can't conceive of starting the day without cereal or toast. But what's wrong with eggs, yogurt, cottage cheese, fruit, ham, or smoked salmon for breakfast? Is it suffering to eat a salad with chicken, tuna lettuce wraps, vegetables with peanut butter, or fruit and cheese for lunch? Is steak and salad, chicken and Brussels sprouts, or salmon and green beans so bad for dinner? Once you are on the plan for a few weeks, you will have no trouble finding a variety of foods to eat.

Wheat, Flour, And Corn Products

After sugar, the most significant bad carbs in our diet are from wheat and corn, typically in bread, pasta, cereal, snack foods, and pastries. Refining whole grains means removing the bran and germ layers, the parts of the grain with fiber, and fiber blunts the rise in glucose. When these layers are removed, it requires even more of the remaining high-glycemic parts of the grain to make bread or whatever product you're making. So, you eat none of the glucose-blunting part and more of the glucose-raising part.

If a food made of wheat is high in carbs to begin with, the worse it is with processing. Whole wheat kernels do not affect blood sugar much. Grinding the wheat and removing the bran and fiber causes the blood sugar to go way up. But it turns out that whole grain flour and similar wholemeal flour have nearly as high a glycemic index despite having none of the bran and fiber removed. This is because there is so much starch in wheat and other grains that we can digest a significant amount of it when the particles are small enough.

Nearly all grains can be processed into flour. Besides the usual wheat flour, you will find rye, barley, and, less commonly, millet and amaranth. These may be slightly better than wheat flour, but the difference isn't enough to help your diet. The popularity of gluten-free products has led to potato and rice flour, even worse than wheat for a low glycemic diet. If it's a gluten-free bakery product, it's likely to be bad for any weight loss plan. Nuts have so little starch and carbohydrates that grinding them into flour or butter has only a minor effect. That is why almond and other nut flours are fine, and all flour from grain is off-limits.

Bread is one of the most challenging things for me to avoid—I grew up on bagels. I don't know anyone who doesn't like bread. It is also very convenient—you can make a lunch or dinner in one minute with bread and lunchmeat. You can make breakfast with two pieces of bread and a toaster. But bread is a significant contributor to our weight problems. White bread has a glycemic index close to 100, as high as pure glucose. In fact, the glycemic index of white bread is higher than eating the equivalent calories of table sugar. It's often used as a standard for the highest possible glycemic index, against which other foods are tested. As we just discussed, whole wheat or whole grain bread is not much better. Some wheat bread in stores has a more modest glycemic index, but they are packed with carbs, meaning you reach the 50-gram limit quickly. Since we cannot moderate very well, we overeat it and ruin our diet. You must avoid all bread if you want to be successful.

Be careful of products labeled "keto bread" or "keto-friendly" bread. A few may be within The Rules—they have no starch, wheat, or sugar; they are made of almond flour and fats. I haven't found any studies examining their effect on blood glucose, but I suppose they would be fine. If you try such a product and notice no change in your weight control, fantastic. A better idea is to make your own. There are many keto sites with recipes. I would recommend one that uses almond flour as the only carb-containing ingredient.

Snack foods are usually made from refined wheat and corn, so you probably can figure out that most such products are forbidden by Rule 2. When in doubt, reading the labels helps. Ritz Crackers, my favorite in the past, have ground wheat, and the label says "wheat flour" right on it. But be careful. The Triscuit label says, "whole grain wheat," and the Wheat Thins label says, "whole grain wheat flour." There may be differences in how the wheat is processed in the delectable snacks, but it doesn't matter. They all have wheat flour, and all must be avoided. Ritz and Wheat Thins have sugar and break Rule 1. I don't even bother reading the labels of crackers and cookies. Virtually all break Rule 1, Rule 2, or both. Don't eat them.

Breakfast cereal is also an effortless meal to prepare. But most cereal is just chopped-up bread or refined corn soaked in a high-sugar sweetener. When I mention the problems with cereal, people are often crestfallen. Yes, most of us like cereal. It's tasty, simple to prepare, and reminds us of childhood. I would be surprised if I've eaten fewer than 500 bowls of Cap'n Crunch cereal. Each bowl was probably two servings. If my estimate is correct, I've eaten over sixty pounds of bad carbs from Cap'n Crunch alone. Even the non-sweet varieties like Cheerios or Shredded Wheat are very high on the glycemic index and will ruin almost any diet. Hot cereals like Cream of Wheat or Malt-O-Meal are the same as cold cereals. All cereal is against The Rules because of the glycemic index and load, and we usually eat far more than a single serving. Put 3/4 cup of cereal into a bowl and see if that is what you typically eat for breakfast.

Pasta is another staple of the American diet. But it's refined wheat with a few other ingredients. It's especially harmful if you're trying to lose weight. The glycemic index isn't all that high, but the serving size is small, and we quickly reach the 50 grams of glycemic index and usually double or triple that with a typical meal. That isn't even counting the junk we put on the pasta. If you could stick to a 2-ounce serving (1/8 of a box) of spaghetti and put no bad carbs on it, you might not gain weight. You might even lose weight. But no one does that. Pasta is off-limits on The Three Rules.

Like bread labeled "keto," there are now "keto" pasta products, often made with bean flour. There are studies showing that chickpea flour has a low glycemic index, but there are no studies on blood sugar with a large meal of chickpea pasta. Until there are such studies, I will avoid it.

Some bean pasta has starch and other additives that may be against Rule 3. If you want to try bean pasta, I recommend you wait until you've been successful on The Rules for at least several weeks. Then, if you add keto pasta, you will know what caused you to stop losing weight.

Most corn products are just as bad as wheat. These include tortillas, cornbread, polenta, grits, and others. Many of these dishes have sugar added, but even without sugar, they are against Rule 2 because they are processed and refined. Refined corn significantly contributes to obesity, but even unrefined corn is problematic because it is starchy, and corn is against Rule 3.

After just a few days on the Three Rules plan, it will be evident that most snack foods and all bread are prohibited. Reading the label will prove it, but be careful. Your default assumption should be not to eat it. Despite what the marketing implies, very few packaged snack foods have truly unprocessed whole grains. If it lists whole wheat berries or another whole grain, and it says unrefined or unprocessed on the package, and I can see the unprocessed, unrefined whole grain in the food, I might eat it. A few snack bars at health food stores fit in this category. But if you can't see the whole grain, assume it's processed and refined. I've said before in this book, and said it nearly every day with patients, "Don't ruin your plans over something that isn't all that good to begin with." Wheat Thins are good, but do you want to sabotage your weight control over them? Would you like to waste all that hard work on a mediocre protein bar? If I go off the diet, give me something better than that, say a Sourdough Jack Burger.

- Do not eat bread or flour from wheat or any grain.
- Do not eat any food made from ground wheat or other grains.
- Do not eat corn products.

Oats

Oats are difficult. As we will learn in Rule 3, all grains have starches that are turned into glucose. Unrefined oats have mostly resistant starches, meaning we don't efficiently digest them into glucose. Most people can eat unrefined oats and still lose weight if they otherwise follow The Rules. The principal problem with oats is when it is made into quick or instant oatmeal or granola. Unrefined oats and other grains are called groats, so unprocessed oats are oat groats. I put oat groats and barley in the same food category; they don't affect blood glucose much, and after cooking, they are very similar in taste.

When I last lost weight, I didn't eat any grains, but now I know that most people can eat unprocessed whole grains (other than corn and rice) and still lose weight. Oat groats are not, however, what you eat when you have oatmeal or granola.

Unprocessed oats can take as long as an hour or longer to cook. Steel-cut oats are groats, chopped into a few pieces, nearly equivalent to groats. Rolled and instant oats are much more refined and can be cooked in a few minutes. The glycemic index rises in processing and refining, with the index of instant oatmeal being about 50% higher than steel-cut oats. I stick to The Rules strictly, so I don't eat any oats except groats and steel-cut. I make large batches of oat groats or barley and add it to yogurt and other foods.[22] It adds texture and tastes great, far better than the packages of instant oatmeal.

While there are some issues with unprocessed whole grains, they are not the primary problem. Quick or instant oatmeal is refined and processed and against The Rules. If your oatmeal was made in a few minutes, it was refined and processed and will interfere with your diet plan. A large bowl of instant oatmeal in the morning ruins many diets, even if you don't add maple syrup and brown sugar.

- Don't eat oatmeal unless it is groats or steel-cut.

Rice

White rice, which is refined and processed, is definitely against Rule 2. It has a high glycemic index, and we frequently eat it excessively. At an Asian restaurant in the United States, people pile white rice on their plates. Even if they choose the entrée without the sweet sauce, their blood glucose will jump, and their weight will rise. White rice will ruin your diet unless you can eat it in insignificant amounts. As always, All or None is easier than moderation. We usually eat the rice in sushi in limited quantities, and some people can lose weight eating it, just as some people can eat a square of chocolate a day. Since I don't do well with even a little of something against The Rules, I don't

---

[22] I make barley by the pasta method rather than what is described on the bag. I put a half-cup or so in a pan, cover it with water, and boil (not simmer) it. In about 20 minutes, it's done. After a few tries, you will know by looking at it.

eat sushi. I recommend avoiding rice entirely for the same reasons that anything against The Rules should be avoided.

Parboiled, also called converted rice, is processed in a way that removes some of the starch and carbohydrates, giving it a lower glycemic index than white rice. But it's still too high on the glycemic load because it's packed with carbs, and you reach 50 grams of the glycemic index in no time. It is tough to moderate, and like all processed, refined foods, it's against Rule 2.

Brown rice (starchy and discussed in the next section) is unprocessed and unrefined, but it has more digestible starches than most unrefined grains and has a high glycemic index and glycemic load. I have seen people substitute brown rice for white rice and overeat it, ruining their diets. I consider all rice to be against The Rules.

Refined grains and the products made from them are high glycemic, difficult to moderate, and addictive in some sense. I would not eat them, sticking entirely to the All or None philosophy. It's too easy to keep going back to the bowl of rice or the all-you-can-eat sushi. Even in small amounts, these foods can ruin diets. Worse, we can't stop at the small amounts.

- Don't eat any rice.

Juice And Refined Fruit Products

Processed and refined wheat causes much of the weight gain in this country. But processed and refined fruit doesn't help. Juice is refined in the terrible sense of the word, having none of the fiber, pulp, or other fruit or vegetable components that slow glucose production.

The other problem with juice is that we drink it quickly. It takes about three oranges to make a cup of juice. We could easily drink a cup of orange juice in a minute, whereas eating three oranges takes time, and I've never eaten three oranges in one sitting. Our blood glucose rises faster and higher than if we ate the whole fruit. Apple, grape, and most other juices are even more problematic because all the fiber and pulp are removed. Even worse, many juices in the store have sugar added, making it even worse for your weight.

All fruit juice is against The Rules, and it is one of the worst things you can consume, nearly as bad as a soft drink. If you see fruit juice in a product's ingredient list, consider it sugar. I don't think I need to tell you, but fruit rolls, candy, and all similar fruit products are against The Rules. They are processed and refined, and they usually have added sugar.

Some vegetable juices, like tomato and carrot juice, might be okay because the sugar content is so low in these vegetables, but I prefer to avoid all juice so I don't have to think about it. I figure there are nearly infinite things that I can eat and drink on this diet, and if I miss a few because The Rules are easier to follow this way, so be it.

I want to comment on smoothies. If you make them yourself in a blender or Vitamix and don't add sugar, that's fine. I only have smoothies at a shop if I am sure there is no sugar added and the whole fruit is in the smoothie. Remember, if pulp and other fruit fiber are removed, then you are drinking juice. Anything else added, such as yogurt, peanut butter, or protein powder, must be free of added sugar or anything else against The Rules.

I eat several servings of fruit a day, and I love it. Eating an apple is more rewarding than drinking apple juice; the same is true for all fruits and vegetables. It makes little sense to ruin your diet over juice or a smoothie when the fruit is better and won't cause weight gain.

- Don't drink juice.
- Don't eat refined fruit products.

Milk and Dairy

It would be nice if Rule Two were perfectly black and white, with all refined foods being bad—it would be easier to remember. A few foods, though, are okay to eat but are technically processed and refined. A stickler would say dairy products such as cheese and yogurt are processed and refined because fat and other milk constituents are removed. But none of what is removed makes a significant difference to your blood sugar or your weight. Milk and dairy products won't cause you to gain weight while on a diet like The Three Rules, and I recommend you eat dairy if you like it.

Multiple studies show that milk and most unsweetened dairy products have a low glycemic index and don't cause weight gain. Unsweetened Greek yogurt is especially good because of all the protein in it. There is no reason on this diet to avoid milk, cheese, or yogurt, whether or not they contain fat. Full-fat dairy products seem to have no ill effects, a fact shown in multiple recent studies. I guess I stick to nonfat yogurt for two reasons. It is inexpensive at Costco, and as my wife reminds me, I still get hung up on what we learned in medical school: all dairy fat is bad, which, as we now know, isn't true. So, my advice is to eat any unsweetened dairy you want. Most yogurt with fruit in it has added sugar, so be careful. Some yogurts will have other additives, and we will talk about them later, but know that some violate Rule 3.

As I mentioned earlier, a superb way to eat yogurt is to put it in a dish or travel container with frozen fruit and leave it in the fridge overnight. I only buy frozen berries. Frozen fruit has all the nutrients of fresh, is typically washed, lasts a long time in the freezer, and is half the price.

- Dairy is good unless there is added sugar or other prohibited additives.

Nut Milks and Other Replacement Milks

Replacement milks made from beans or nuts, such as soy, almond, coconut, cashew, macadamia, and others, are allowed in The Three Rules. These milks are made by grinding the nuts or beans, adding water, and removing some byproducts. This is another case where some refining doesn't make a difference.

I drank unsweetened almond milk for a long time before realizing that it was technically refined by my definition. I looked into the various milks, and although some of the nut is removed, the glycemic index doesn't change much from the index of the original form. Also, since a cup of the drink is mostly water, there are so few carbs in it that the glycemic load is negligible. For example, a cup of unsweetened almond milk has one gram of carbohydrates and no sugar. Remember that the glycemic index is calculated from 50 grams of carbohydrates, so 50 cups of almond milk would be needed. A cup of the drink doesn't make a difference. Would I prefer that The Three Rules were perfect and there were no "good" foods that technically violate the wording of The Rules? Yes. But nature and life are imperfect. If you want to be an absolute Three Rules purist, avoid all the replacement milks and stick with whole dairy milk. But over the years, I have improved at making peace with imperfection, so I drink almond milk.

All the replacement milks listed above are fine, but don't drink rice or oat milk. Most rice milk is made from white rice or highly refined rice flour. Some are chemically (enzymatically) processed, and the starches are converted to sugar—even worse. The important thing is that the glycemic index of rice milk is much higher than that of regular milk or nut milk. A cup of rice milk has about 25 grams of carbohydrates, meaning that in contrast to almond milk, with its one gram of carbohydrates per cup, with rice milk, you're halfway to the 50-gram carb level of the glycemic index. Don't drink it.

Oat milk is similarly against The Rules. The oats are refined to make the milk, and often, the starches are treated with enzymes to make the oats more digestible, producing sugar in the process. Oat milk may not list sugar in the ingredients, but some brands have added sugars in the Nutrition Facts section. The FDA considers sugar created by this method to be added, just like the sugar added to soda.[23] Either way, oat milk is refined, and like instant oats, it is against Rule 2.

---

[23] https://www.fda.gov/regulatory-information/search-fda-guidance-documents/guidance-industry-nutrition-and-supplement-facts-labels-questions-and-answers-related-compliance

Tofu is made by coagulating soy milk in much the same way that cheese is made from regular milk. In some health food stores, you will see non-dairy "cheese" made similarly from nuts and other beans. Just like dairy cheese, these are all fine.

As always, you must read the labels if you drink replacement milk or eat cheese made from it. Most drinks at the store have added sugar, and a few have prohibited food additives. (We'll discuss food additives more in the Rule 3 section.) Obviously, sugar breaks Rule 1—No Added Sugar. I never drink soy or almond milk at a restaurant or coffee shop without reading the label. The coffee shops will usually let you see the package, and in most cases, sugar is added. If I want something to lighten my coffee at a restaurant, I use milk or cream— I have never seen sugar added to these. Of course, whipped cream may have sugar added. Unfortunately, Reddi-Whip, the delicious whipped cream you can spray onto anything, has sugar and corn syrup added.

- Unsweetened replacement milk from soy or nuts is fine.
- Do not drink rice milk.

Alcohol

We all know that alcohol has significant health risks and can affect one's ability to lose weight. Alcohol is made from carbohydrates, so we must discuss it in Rule 2. Alcohol's effect on health and weight is confusing and controversial. People have strong opinions on how much we should drink, how much is safe, and even the morality of drinking. I will try to stick to the facts, but my opinion may show through. Beer is against Rule 2 because it has refined grain, usually wheat or barley. Sweetened drinks, including sweet wines, have sugar added and are against Rule 1. Dry wine is made from grape juice, but the sugar is consumed by yeast. Hard liquor, such as whiskey or vodka, has no carbs and is within The Rules.

Some studies show that alcohol in moderation can lower the risk of heart disease. I have concerns about the validity of these studies because they were not randomized and prospective. The people in the control groups, those who do not drink at all, may have quit because of health problems or previous heavy alcohol use, potentially affecting the study's conclusions. I am confident, though, that no one should drink alcohol to improve their health. Many people cannot drink in moderation, and when consumed in larger quantities (more than a drink a day for women or two a day for men), alcohol is clearly harmful, increasing the risk of liver disease, heart problems, stroke, and cancer. We all know the dangers of acute intoxication, and many Americans can't consume alcohol without risking binging or becoming addicted. I will put all that aside for now and discuss the effects of alcohol on a carbohydrate-based diet.

Alcohol has variable effects on glucose metabolism, depending on the person and when they drink it. An important factor is what type of alcoholic drink you consume. Beer contributes to weight gain, presumably by raising glucose,[24] and most heavy beer drinkers I know are overweight or obese. Studies are less conclusive with dry

---

[24] Sluik D, Atkinson FS, Brand-Miller JC, Fogelholm M, Raben A, Feskens EJ. Contributors to dietary glycaemic index and glycaemic load in the Netherlands: the role of beer. Br J Nutr. 2016;115(7):1218-1225. doi:10.1017/S0007114516000052

wine and spirits, though alcohol in any form in high quantities can raise blood sugar for some people.[25]

If you want to lose weight, you shouldn't drink beer, sweet wine, or cocktails with added sugar. If you drink dry wine or liquor, you are within The Three Rules, but too much of either could sabotage your diet plans and possibly your life plans. If you cannot drink in moderation, you have three problems. First, you may not lose weight because of the effects of alcohol on your metabolism. Second, you are more likely to make poor food choices, not to mention many other poor decisions. And third, you probably should abstain from alcohol entirely since if you can't drink in moderation, you, by definition, have an alcohol problem.

- Do not drink beer.
- Do not drink sweet wine.
- Dry wine and liquor are within The Rules, but be careful.

---

[25] Hätönen KA, Virtamo J, Eriksson JG, et al. Modifying effects of alcohol on the postprandial glucose and insulin responses in healthy subjects. Am J Clin Nutr. 2012;96(1):44-49. doi:10.3945/ajcn.111.031682

Rule Three:
Do Not Eat Starchy Vegetables or Fruits, Especially Potatoes, Corn, And Rice

As you recall from the initial chapters, starch is a carbohydrate molecule broken down into sugar. Many starches, especially those in potatoes, are digested quickly into glucose, causing all the problems with weight that we've discussed. We love potatoes, and we eat a lot in many forms. Ironically, the classic meat and potatoes diet causes more harm from the potatoes than the meat. If you eliminate potatoes from your diet, you have almost mastered this rule.

Don't get hung up on botanical terms. I used to be concerned about whether a tomato is a fruit, whether grains are fruits, and whether corn is a grain, a fruit, or a vegetable. Who cares? I call all nuts "nuts," whether they are tree nuts, legumes, or something else. Corn is a vegetable in some settings and a grain or cereal in others. As far as this diet goes, it doesn't matter. Starchy is starchy, and we should avoid it whether it's a starchy fruit, vegetable, grain, or combination.

Not all starches are problematic. The starch in potatoes is easily digested and converted to glucose. Others are not as easily digested and are called resistant starches. The list of foods with a considerable amount of starch is long, and most consist of resistant starches and don't matter to us. Beans and other legumes, squash, and nuts have mostly resistant starches and are great to eat; I don't think of these as starchy foods. For the purpose of the Rule, they are not starchy—we only care about the easily digestible starches, the ones that cause us to gain weight. Beans and nuts are good, and I eat them almost every day. Potatoes, sweet potatoes, corn, and rice have too much digestible starch; they are starchy and against Rule 3. A few foods are in a gray area and have variable amounts of resistant and digestible starches, depending on how you eat them—bananas are the most significant.

In this chapter, I will review the most important fruits and vegetables, elaborate on grains, and discuss a few more food additives. But if all you take home is the fundamental point of Rule 3, you will do well. Do not eat potatoes, sweet potatoes, corn, or rice.

- Beans, nuts, and most fruits and vegetables are good.
- Do not eat potatoes, sweet potatoes, corn, or rice.

Potatoes

I love potatoes. I have known very few people who do not enjoy eating potatoes in one form or another. They are inexpensive and give us quick energy. Unfortunately, everything comes with a price. The potato has a high glycemic index because of its rapidly digestible starch and is the prototype of a starchy vegetable. It's difficult to lose weight if you eat potatoes, even if you almost starve yourself the rest of the day.

Years ago, Americans could get by with a potato at dinner because, as we've discussed, our lives differed in what we ate and the energy we burned with everyday activities. Meat and potatoes at dinner would sustain us. The meat gave us protein and fat, and the potato supplied all the needed carbs. A few green vegetables and fruit once in a while, and we were good. Now, we eat potatoes in multiple forms all the time. Chips, fries, mashed, hash browns, baked, boiled—it doesn't matter. It's all high glycemic and bad for any diet. We were told long ago that what you put on a baked potato, such as sour cream or bacon, caused the weight gain. That isn't true, at least not now. In our current situation, it is the glucose generated from the potato itself.

Potatoes have health benefits, as almost anything has benefits and harms. But potatoes, in the context of the current American diet, contribute to weight gain. If you could stick to a low-calorie, low-glycemic diet, as nearly everyone did a hundred years ago, you could eat some potatoes and not gain weight.

Potatoes also act like an addictive substance. I am sure they aren't truly addictive like a drug, but once you get started, like so many tasty carbs, it's difficult to stop. Just like in the old Lay's potato chip commercial, it is hard to eat just one. I find it relatively easy to have none, but not one. If you cannot give up potatoes entirely, you will not lose weight on The Three Rules. If you give them up and follow Rules 1 and 2, you will lose weight.

- Do not eat potatoes in any form.

Sweet Potatoes and Other Root Vegetables

The first question people ask me after I talk about potatoes is, "What about sweet potatoes?" We love sweet potatoes (sometimes called yams) but don't eat them nearly as often as white potatoes. We eat more now because people realize potatoes cause weight gain, so they try to get by with sweet potatoes. It doesn't work. Sweet potatoes are starchy and have a high glycemic index and glycemic load. They are addictive, making the All or None approach best. Think of sweet potatoes as potatoes—they are against The Rules.

Few other root vegetables concern us. Many low-carb diets list beets as a food to be avoided. If they are canned or pickled, sugar is often added, but if no sugar is added, you can eat them; beets aren't starchy enough to be a problem. No one got fat on beets. The key difference between beets and sweet potatoes is that beets have far less starch. The glycemic load of beets is one-third that of sweet potatoes. Carrots are also sometimes on "do not eat" lists. Forget it. Carrots have almost no carbs and very little sugar. Parsnips, turnips, and kohlrabi (which I do not recall ever eating) are other root vegetables of no concern. Rutabagas, yucca, and cassava (tapioca) are starchy and should be avoided. Fortunately, that is easy to do.

- Do not eat sweet potatoes.
- Rutabaga, yucca, and cassava are no good either.

Corn

We talked about products made from processed, refined corn, which are definitely against The Rules. What about whole corn, either as sweet corn or as popcorn?

Sweet corn is against Rule 3. It's starchy and will raise your glucose. It may not raise your sugar as much as potato, gram for gram, but again, the All or None approach is best. I can easily go back for a second or third ear of corn or another bowl of a sweet corn side dish. In The Three Rules, you don't want to eat anything where moderation is critical. The glycemic load of corn is not that high, but that relies on serving size. There are 3.5 servings of corn in a typical can. If I could stick to one serving, I wouldn't have needed to lose weight so many times. I don't pick out stray kernels of corn in a restaurant salad, but I don't order a side dish of corn.

Popcorn is the only other unprocessed corn product to consider. It's starchy like all corn, but given the air in the popcorn, a serving size is relatively low in carbohydrates. For that reason, many carb-based diets will allow popcorn, <u>but I don't recommend it and consider it against The Rules</u>. It's addictive, will raise your glucose, and will interfere with your diet. When your glucose rises, the butter you put on the popcorn and the oil you used to make it worsen the problem. I find Rule 3 simple: No starchy fruits or vegetables, especially potatoes, corn, and rice. All corn is off-limits under Rule 3.

- Do not eat corn.
- Processed and refined corn products are especially against The Rules.

Rice And Whole Grains

As I have mentioned, not every food or every food group is either great for the diet or bad for it, black or white. Grains are the most significant gray area. Refined grains are part of Rule 2, and I discuss whole grains now in Rule 3, knowing that some readers will tell me grains are not fruits or vegetables. Fine, I accept it, but that is semantics. I don't care what you call them.

Due to refining and processing, white rice and its products are against Rule 2. Brown rice is a gray area food because it has a moderate glycemic index and glycemic load. It has more digestible starch than oats, barley, and most other grains; therefore, its glycemic load is higher. It's also difficult to eat any rice in moderation. When you make it at home, you must be very careful not to overeat it. Since it has that potential, you are far better off not eating brown rice. <u>Consider all rice to be against Rule 3.</u> It's not worth sacrificing your diet and weight for rice.

I want to clarify an aspect of the Three Rules. The Rules prohibits bad carbs. In most instances, that means that the glycemic index or load is high, where one serving will cause a problem. Some foods, such as brown rice, may not have a high glycemic load, but they are addictive. Since it is so difficult to eat in small amounts, we eat far more carbs than the 50 grams of the glycemic index, ruining our diet. These foods, including all rice, are against The Rules.

Some people can eat brown rice without a problem. They will continue to lose weight, and when they reach their goal, they can eat brown rice and not regain weight. I am not such a person. I don't recommend it, but if you want to try brown rice, be very careful. If your weight doesn't come off as expected, or if you start to regain what you lost, blame it on the brown rice and stop eating it. Rule 3 works best for most of us—do not eat starchy vegetables and fruits, especially potatoes, corn, and rice. I recommend that if you try eating brown rice, put additional wording into Rule 3 for yourself, something like "Do not eat starchy vegetables or fruits, especially potatoes, corn, and white rice—brown rice is fine." Call it a Rule 3 Variation. Maybe it will work for you, but you still need an ironclad Rule to follow. You don't want to accumulate ambiguous exceptions to The Rules. Remember, one of the essential parts of The Rules is that it's All or None. I don't recommend eating brown rice, but your Rule Variation may work for you.

Other than rice, the other grains, if unprocessed, are acceptable. I discussed oats extensively with Rule 2—unprocessed oat groats and steel-cut oats have more resistant than digestible starches, and the glycemic index and load are low, so they are fine. Barley, quinoa, wheat berries, farro, and nearly all other unprocessed, non-rice grains are fine. Virtually all wheat products are refined and processed and against Rule 2. Wheat berries, occasionally seen in health food stores, are wheat groats and are unprocessed. Wheat berries are fine, but make sure you see the whole grain in the food and that it isn't refined wheat or wheat berry flour.

Avoid all rice, corn, and processed wheat, which is almost all the wheat you will see in food. If you come across a grain you don't know, search for its glycemic load. If it's similar to quinoa and barley and is unprocessed and unrefined, eat it if you want. Again, except for rice, most unprocessed grains are acceptable in The Three Rules, but you can't be ridiculous. Don't test The Rules by eating a pound of hulled barley in one sitting. You don't have to moderate or measure acceptable grains, but don't be ridiculous.

I spent a lot of time talking about grains, probably more than necessary, and I don't want you to worry about it much. Stick with The Rules, and you will be fine. Rule Three is straightforward. Avoiding potatoes, corn, rice, and a few other foods is all it takes.

- Do not eat rice of any kind.
- Do not eat any ground or processed wheat.
- All other whole grains are fine, but don't be ridiculous.

Bananas

Bananas and plantains are the only fruits worth mentioning that have significant digestible starch. I sometimes say that no one got fat eating bananas. While that is almost certainly true, bananas have a lot of starch, so we need to discuss them. If you stick to the absolute Rules and the All or None approach, then don't eat bananas. Plantains and unripe bananas have relatively resistant starch, and the glycemic index is reasonably low. Ripe bananas and plantains have a higher glycemic index and glycemic load. Banana chips and fried plantains have the highest glycemic load and are addictive. Avoid them completely.

I will occasionally eat bananas, but only if they are on the green side. If you want to do that, feel free. If you decide that bananas aren't worth eating, don't eat them. I would not eat ripe or overripe bananas, but I have never seen people gain weight on bananas, and people usually don't develop a habit of overeating them. If you eat bananas frequently, try the less ripe ones. I may be drawing too thin a line of distinction, and I don't think your success will hinge on the decision about bananas, regardless of the ripeness of the bananas you enjoy. If you notice, the Rule reads "especially potatoes, corn, and rice" because they are the only starchy vegetables or fruits we eat regularly enough to make much difference. If you are one of the few who eat lots of ripe bananas, cassava, or yucca, you will have to make a change.

- Be careful with ripe bananas.
- Do not eat banana chips or fried plantains.

Squash

There are many types of squash. The summer squashes are zucchini and the classic yellow squash. Winter squashes are spaghetti, acorn, butternut, pumpkin, and related varieties. Summer squash is less starchy than winter squash, but even the winter varieties have much less digestible starch than potatoes, sweet potatoes, corn, or rice. Spaghetti squash, lately becoming more popular, is especially low glycemic. All squash varieties have an appreciable amount of fiber, do not raise blood glucose much, and won't affect your weight loss plan. I don't consider any squash to be starchy. Eat squash if you want, summer or winter; just don't add brown sugar.

Starchy Food Additives

Not many foods are prohibited by Rule 3—mainly potatoes, sweet potatoes, corn, and rice. You must also avoid packaged and prepared foods that use starch from fruits and vegetables, so read the labels. Even some yogurt and replacement milks have these additives. It's obvious when the ingredient list includes corn starch that you shouldn't eat it. Adding corn starch to a sauce is worse than eating the corn itself. (Don't eat sauce with flour added either.) But what about tapioca, maltodextrin, or other additives?

Tapioca is starch from cassava. It's a common additive, especially in gluten-free products. Maltodextrin is a starch from various plants. Don't eat either. Occasionally, there is something on a label I have never heard of; I look it up, and it's a starch. Look up words until you know the names of all the food starches. This is just like Rule One, where you have to learn the dozens of words for sugar. Fortunately, most of us have smartphones and internet access, and you can quickly look a word up in the store.

Remember, All or None is the best approach. Since there is no way to tell just how much corn starch is added when it's on the label, don't eat it. There are many other things to eat. The same holds true with restaurants or other settings when you don't make the food. I was at a party recently and was told there were no carbs in a stew. We were chatting, and I saw someone dumping corn starch into it without measuring how much he was using. Would eating that have killed me? Of course not. But why ruin a diet with corn starch? I'd rather have an ear of corn or a Sourdough Jack Burger. So, find out what is in your food and eat with intent. Don't eat starchy fruits or vegetables, and don't eat foods prepared with starch from them.

Part 4

Common Questions and Misconceptions

Sometimes, simple things appear complicated, and vice versa.

Over the years, I have seen people fail due to minor errors or misunderstandings of The Rules. I'll discuss some of these common mistakes and other tips that will help you succeed and repeat some important pointers I made earlier. It's a terrible feeling to fail at a diet or any plan over a simple misunderstanding. If you stray from the diet, make it count, enjoy it, and get back to work. Don't ruin the plan over something simple, avoidable, and unenjoyable.

How Strict Are the Rules?

*Succeeding at something important always takes
hard work and discipline. If that is being strict,
I accept it.*

A theme throughout this book has been how easy it is to gain weight and how difficult it is to lose it. You cannot lose weight without work. That is a simple, undeniable fact. Trying to find wiggle room to keep eating something you like rarely works. It's up to you to decide if it's worth the work required. Giving up some foods you like is a big deal, but there are still countless appetizing foods on the Three Rules. I don't eat tofu and broccoli all day long. I promise.

You may be lucky. You may find that you can follow The Rules 90% and still succeed. Most people can't. I can't. I have come to grips with the reality that I cannot go outside The Rules and keep my weight in control. Perhaps I could get away with one Sourdough Jack Burger monthly or one bagel and cream cheese every other Sunday. But I have failed many times trying things like that. There may be recovering alcohol abusers who can drink on the first day of every month. For every such person, I would bet a hundred relapse after that one drink.

All Or None and All In

I have discussed the All or None philosophy of the Three Rules more times than you want to hear. I believe that All or None is what makes this diet work for most people. Other diets cut back on bad carbs, but the failure rate of these diets is high because you have to moderate your intake. Moderation takes willpower. Eating one Thin Mint cookie, a few french fries, or one Lindor chocolate truffle is difficult. Not having even a taste of something? That, to me, is easier. I take pride in it and have a sense of accomplishment. I feel the same way when I don't have a glass of the wine everyone else is drinking. If I don't have one, I can't have two and wake up with regret and a headache. One treat often leads to two. Zero never leads to one, and so two is impossible. People say alcohol is not a fair comparison. They say you don't have to drink, but you do have to eat. That is a fallacy. You do have to drink, but you don't have to drink alcohol. You do have to eat, but you don't have to eat added sugar, processed and refined carbs, or starchy fruits or vegetables.

I recommended The Three Rules to patients every day. At my peak, I saw twenty patients daily (since the first edition, I cut back and am now retired). About twelve were there for routine visits, and I recommended The Three Rules five or six times. Each time I recommended The Rules, I told them to start only if they were committed. You must be All In. I advised them to put all their effort into it. I only recommended All or None. You will succeed if you go All In and eat All or None. If you do not, you may fail. You will probably fail.

All or None refers to the fact that you can eat all you want within The Rules if you eat none of what is against The Rules. Yes, if you eat buckets of fruit at a time (see later in this section), you could overwhelm your body's ability to handle the sugar and gain weight. But that scenario is so rare that I don't worry about it. Much more common than eating buckets of fruit is eating a cookie or two or a small bowl of ice cream. A cookie or a little ice cream isn't *none*. Ice cream and cookies will ruin almost any diet. One sample at Costco leads to several; one ear of corn leads to two; one Hershey's Kiss leads to a bowl.

I recently explained The Rules to a patient. They said they already did it because they didn't eat much bread. Please do not think that way. Not eating much does not mean anything. First, who defines "much?" Second, as we've discussed, the human body is very good at storing fat from just a little extra energy. It doesn't take "much" bread or sugar to ruin your diet. None—that works. It is easier to follow, and it takes less willpower. If you asked an alcoholic you love if they drank today, you would never want the answer to be, "Not much."

This diet plan is not for everyone, but it works if you do it. Only start The Three Rules plan if you are All In. If you want to succeed in anything, that is your best chance. Devote all your energy to the Three Rules, and you will succeed. That philosophy holds true in so many things: learning a language, succeeding in your job, and doing well in school. You will succeed if you focus, devote all your efforts, and go All In.

Can You Still Enjoy Eating?

Can you still enjoy eating? With near certainty, you will enjoy eating more. You will have to give up the immediate pleasure of Rocky Road ice cream, but you will gain the more profound joy of control over what you eat. How many times have you woken up regretting the amount of unhealthy food you ate the day before? Have you ever felt good about yourself after overeating fast food? Eating healthy is like exercise. You will feel good after having done it. Feeling good about yourself is the best enjoyment there is.

Sure, but will you enjoy eating? I know that is a different question. I only eat food I enjoy. I regularly eat steak, ham, chicken, salmon, shrimp, pork roast, and all kinds of soups, and I enjoy them all. We eat plenty of vegetables—roasted, steamed, and sautéed, all with delicious sauces. Apples, oranges, grapefruit, berries, cheese, cold cuts, and eggs. I can go on and on.

My wife, who has not had a weight problem, enjoys our meals. (I do most of the cooking, and while it's possible she's fibbing a bit, she has yet to kick me out of the kitchen.) When our son was home from college, he ate with us most nights and never went to McDonald's with his friends after an unfinished meal. In fact, his friends have told him that the dinners they have had at our house are some of the best meals they've ever eaten. We just returned from a vacation and ate out every meal—I enjoyed them all.

Since I went All In on The Rules about seven years ago, I have been essentially All or None. The rare times I went off the plan, I did it deliberately, with intent, for a 50th-anniversary party or some other special event. I have not woken up regretting what I had eaten the day before. Not a single time. That is a beautiful feeling, making me want to work hard every day.

I want you to experience the same enjoyment. If you continue what you are doing now or start The Rules or another diet plan and fail because you aren't strict enough, you will feel bad about yourself. Then, you definitely will not enjoy eating, at least not for longer than a few minutes.

Cheat Days

Many diets allow or even recommend cheat days. This is when you "cheat" on your diet once a week, once a month, or whatever. Based on my All or None philosophy, you probably figured out I am against cheat days. First, I don't like the word "cheat" in this situation. I am happy with The Three Rules; I am proud that I have been on it for several years; I am pleased with the success it has brought me, and I am enjoying my life more. If I ate a Sourdough Jack Burger, I would be cheating myself, hurting myself.

Most of us will not stop at one cheat day a week or a month. It often leads to more and more straying from the diet. This is precisely why Alcoholics Anonymous doesn't recommend a cheat day of drinking, drug counselors rarely recommend a cheat day for heroin, and no one recommends a cheat day in your marriage. Let us decide how we want to live and stick with it the best we can. Do I ever eat anything off The Rules? It's rare, but it happens. But when I eat something against The Rules, I do it happily, with intent, not cheating anyone or anything. And then, immediately after, I am back with The Rules.

You Cannot Be Ridiculous

Human beings can gain weight without bad carbs. We could probably gain weight with no carbs. If you ate enough pure protein, fat, or good carbs and did it quickly enough, you might overwhelm your ability to control the glucose rise. You might gain weight. In my experience, this is very difficult and uncommon. Most people would fill up and stop eating before their glucose rose too high since protein and fat suppress appetite. When people gain weight, it is almost always from bad carbs.

I tell people they can eat what they want unless it's against The Rules. You don't need to measure foods or count carbs. You can eat three apples or a pound of shrimp. But if you go crazy, eating ridiculous amounts, say, a 60-ounce steak or several pounds of shrimp soaked in butter, then I am not so sure you would still lose weight that day. Doing that is ridiculous. I criticize myself when I "eat from the trough." By this, I mean sitting next to a bowl or bag of food and eating from it all day. That is not a recipe for success, though if the food is within The Rules, you might be okay. My point is this: eat what you want, but don't be ridiculous, and don't eat from the trough.

What About Protein and Fat?

If you eat something without carbohydrates,
did you really eat it?

The Three Rules affects only what you eat that has carbohydrates—sugar, processed and refined carbs, and starchy foods. Protein and fats have no sugar, no starch, and no carbs at all. If all you ate were protein and fats, you would lose weight unless you were ridiculous or ate all day from the trough. This is the basis of the ketogenic and Atkins diets. (As you recall, I don't recommend these diets because people eventually go off the diets and regain their weight quickly.)

Since we are not eliminating all carbohydrates, can you still eat all the protein and fat you want and lose weight? If you are strict with The Rules, you can. All protein and fat are neutral if you stay within The Three Rules. They do not help, and they do not hurt. Since you give up bad carbs when obeying the Three Rules, you have to eat something else. Protein, fat, and good carbs are what you choose from—that is all there is. Fortunately, all three categories can be delicious.

If you don't follow The Rules closely, protein and fat will add to your weight gain. A hamburger bun by itself, clearly against The Rules, is bad enough. If you put a double cheeseburger with mayo on it, you will not lose weight, and the extra calories will cause you to gain weight. Calories from fat, protein, and carbs matter. They matter much, much more if you eat the bad carbs. If you don't eat the bun or anything else against The Rules, you will lose weight, even if you eat the double cheeseburger. There are a few other issues about protein and fat, but they are straightforward.

Meats And Fish

Since you will give up bad carbs, you'll eat good carbs, protein, and fat. Unless you are a vegan, much of the protein will be red meat, poultry, and fish, with some from nuts, beans, and vegetables. Vegans get all their protein from plants—more difficult but achievable. As I just said, meats and fish, having no carbs, are always fine on The Three Rules. If you cave in and eat bad carbs, you will gain weight from the protein and fat in anything you eat. If you do not eat bad carbs, you won't.

Be careful of a few things when eating meat and fish. Eating it at home is easy. Don't put anything on it that has sugar, processed and refined carbs, or starchy fruit and vegetables. When you eat out, or if you eat from a package, you have to watch out. If there is a label, read it. Beef jerky and cold cuts often have added sugar and starch, many sauces have outlawed foods, and most fried foods will have breading. If you are out for a meal, and there is no label, ask what is in it. If in doubt, don't eat it. Ask for sauce on the side, no sauce, or whatever you have to do. Don't let breading on the chicken or sauce on the shrimp ruin your plans. Don't just eat it because it's there.

If it's your mother's fried chicken, and you want to eat it, that is up to you. But if you eat it, do so knowing that you are going against your plans and that it will affect your diet. Eat it with intent. Then start back with The Rules again, right after the meal. Eating the leftovers the following day is probably not worth it and could begin a habit.

Fats and Oils

Fats and oils are simple. If you only eat within The Rules, then they don't matter. If you eat bad carbs, then fats and oils make it worse. Certain fats are better for you than others for health reasons but not for weight loss. Though there is no absolute consensus, olive and canola oil seem to be excellent for heart health. Perhaps cold-pressed canola is better than commercially refined, but it can be hard to find. Lately, I have been using cold-pressed avocado oil for its healthy fats and high smoke point. These choices have nothing to do with weight loss, but if I use oil, I find the healthiest.

I am still unsure about coconut oil and see no need to eat it. Most other plant-derived oils are fine for heart health, and again, no oils will interfere with the Three Rules.

Meat and dairy fats may not be as good for you as plant oils, but they are not as harmful as previously thought. In fact, dairy products, especially yogurt and cheese, may lower the risk of cardiovascular disease and diabetes. Unless there is added sugar or other off-limits food additives, all dairy is within The Rules. Read the label, and it's easy.

Eggs

Eggs have no carbohydrates, are an excellent source of protein, and fill us up for the day. Whole eggs or egg whites are the same under The Three Rules. It should go without saying by now that you must know what else is in the egg dish. Most omelets have no added sugar or processed and refined carbs, but ask or read the label of everything you eat. Clearly, if potatoes are on the side or in the egg dish itself, then it's against The Rules.

Unrelated to weight loss, the media and websites have recently droned on how eggs are good for you. Eating eggs in moderation has little risk if a person is at low risk of coronary heart disease. But, if someone has a heart problem or is at high risk of a heart attack, they should talk to their doctor and probably cut back on eggs. I buy egg whites in cartons at Costco; it's inexpensive and simple to make into an omelet or scrambled eggs. I will leave the issue of eggs and heart risk to you and your doctor, but eggs are fine as far as The Three Rules is concerned.

Addiction To Bad Carbs

Since writing the first edition, I have changed my thinking about addiction. First, I do not consider sugar or other bad carbs to be nearly as addictive as heroin, alcohol, or other drugs. My distinction is whether we abstain from a substance by accident, without conscious thought. We think we are addicted to treats but often skip them because we are out of town or the Dunkin' Donuts is closed. A heroin addict never misses a day of heroin use because something comes up. They will do everything possible to get a new supply. Bad carbs have a pull on us, but they are not as addictive as drugs. You'll notice that I still use the adjective addictive for simplicity.

The more significant change in my thoughts on addiction is a concept called harm reduction. My first exposure to the idea was in

Maia Szalavitz's superb book, *Undoing Drugs*. She writes primarily about opiates, but the concept applies to all addictions and non-addictive substances we struggle to avoid. With opiates such as heroin, most agree that complete abstinence is the best long-term solution. But that is unfeasible or impossible for many people. Interventions other than abstinence can reduce harm while not completely solving the problem.

For example, allowing nurse-supervised heroin use, while controversial, can lower the risk of overdose and allow some highly motivated users to live more normal lives rather than commit crimes to make money to fuel their secret problem. Ms. Szalavitz's book made me realize there may be benefits to cutting back on bad carbs instead of the all-or-none approach of eliminating them entirely. I still believe that if your goal, your "end in mind," is to be fit and thin, strictly following The Three Rules is the answer. But for some, it is too stressful, and with that approach, they fail entirely. Cutting back on bad carbs can reduce harm by helping people lose some weight, and the diet has health benefits independent of weight loss. A normal weight, achievable with The Three Rules, is better than remaining overweight or mildly obese. But losing some weight is better than losing none. That is the concept of harm reduction. I advise you to commit to my All or None approach and strictly embrace The Three Rules. But if you make an honest attempt and find it impossible, following The Rules the best you can will reduce the harm of being obese or overweight.

Special Topics

A few things need further explanation.

The media, the internet, and people you know cannot always be trusted. The problem is that much of what they say is true, but some is entirely false. This is the case in every aspect of life, and diets are no exception. You will hear claims about what is missing from a diet like The Three Rules, unhealthy foods that should not be allowed, and foods that The Rules allows that may raise blood sugar. There will be websites talking about a harmful food additive, and you will see ads and medical sites claiming that there is food that will burn fat. I will explain a few of these topics, but there is no reason for controversy. The Rules allows for various approaches—you can follow the plan if you disagree with my opinions about health, if you are a vegan, if you keep kosher, if you only eat organic food, or if you have no dietary restrictions. Just don't eat foods against The Rules.

Remember that The Three Rules is designed to help you lose weight, not to solve every health problem. If there is food within The Rules that you feel is harmful, don't eat it. If you miss out on one or two otherwise healthy foods, try not to worry about it. The Three Rules allows for so much variety that this won't be an issue.

Is The Three Rules Diet Healthy?

We have discussed how The Three Rules will solve your weight problem. We know that bad carbs cause obesity, and eliminating them results in weight loss. Some still believe that cutting carbs, even bad carbs, is unhealthy. I don't want to belabor the point—there are many, many studies showing the health benefits of eliminating sugar and refined carbohydrates. I was not going to write this section, but a study this month confirmed for the umpteenth time the cardiovascular benefits of cutting out bad carbs.[26] This study should put to rest any further concerns about a low glycemic index diet and, by extension, The Three Rules. After twelve months, improving one's diet with respect to sugar and refined carbohydrates improved blood pressure, body weight, waist circumference, fasting glucose, hemoglobin A1C (a measure of overall glucose levels), triglycerides, and cholesterol.

We already know that losing weight helps with all the medical problems associated with obesity. It's also clear that losing weight on The Three Rules by eliminating bad carbs directly benefits the factors that contribute to cardiovascular disease. If anyone tries to say otherwise, this study and a simple internet search should satisfy them. If you look hard enough, you can find the downsides and risks to anything. You could catch influenza at a movie theater, fall and break your hip at the grocery store, and get in an accident anytime

---

[26] Martínez-González MA, Fernandez-Lazaro CI, Toledo E, et al. Carbohydrate quality changes and concurrent changes in cardiovascular risk factors: a longitudinal analysis in the PREDIMED-Plus randomized trial. Am J Clin Nutr. 2020;111(2):291-306. doi:10.1093/ajcn/nqz298

you drive. Do not let negative people and saboteurs convince you to keep eating bad carbs because they find a minor problem with The Three Rules.

Aren't There Healthy Foods Against the Rules and Unhealthy Foods That Obey the Rules?

Most foods within The Rules are also good for us for reasons other than weight control. Fruits, vegetables, beans, nuts, dairy, lean meats, fish, and chicken are all healthy and are fine on the Three Rules plan. Most foods against The Rules, such as pastries, other sweets, pasta, bread, and cereal, are unhealthy or at least not especially good for us. There are exceptions. On The Rules, you won't eat a few otherwise healthy foods, such as brown rice and corn. I accept it. There will always be healthy foods you don't eat. There are hundreds of fruits and vegetables that you won't eat because they are unavailable where you live or you don't like them. One trip down the aisle at an Indian market (one of my favorite places to shop), and you will realize you have never heard of most beans and vegetables that exist. You can never eat all the healthy foods. If you miss out on a few because they are against The Rules, so be it. Overall, you will be much healthier after losing weight.

I want to comment on the word "healthy." Right before I retired, I mentioned to a diabetic patient that they should give up potatoes to help with weight loss and lower their glucose readings. They said they thought potatoes were healthy. Healthy is an ambiguous term. Like most foods, potatoes have good and bad properties. If you are looking for tasty, inexpensive nutrition, potatoes are great. The potato has been beneficial in the past when food was scarce. Potatoes have vitamins that we need to live. But if you have a weight problem, then potatoes are not healthy. Many foods are like that. Breakfast cereal has vitamins and fiber. It is only unhealthy if you want to lower your blood sugars and lose weight.

Most things in life have upsides and downsides. A car is vital if you need to drive to work. Yet we all know that there are thousands of severe car accidents yearly. Try to think about the benefits and negatives of all foods. Is eating food outside The Rules, if healthy in some ways, worth the downsides? Is one health benefit worth the negative effect on your weight? Since obesity is one of the leading causes of morbidity and mortality, I would rather you lose weight and find another way to get the health benefits provided by potatoes or any food that is against The Rules.

Two analogies to giving up some healthy foods to lose weight are allergy and alcohol (again). Nuts are good for you, but if you are allergic, the health benefits of nuts are clearly outweighed by the negatives. Shellfish, milk, and strawberries are healthy foods to which people are often allergic. You would never advise someone to eat them anyway. Alcohol may have a few health benefits, but an alcoholic or someone with liver disease is advised not to drink alcohol, regardless of the possible benefits. I think of bad carbs the same way. Sure, there are some benefits to a few foods that are against The Rules. Don't eat them—the downside is too great.

There are also some iffy or downright unhealthy foods that are within The Rules. Trans-fat, the worst food additive, which used to be in margarine and shortening, is within The Rules, as are all fats. Processed red meat has health risks. But this is a book about weight. I recommended that my patients avoid trans-fat, minimize processed red meat, and choose fish and poultry over unprocessed red meat, though red meat is not as bad as we thought for many years. Eating a lot of eggs if you have a history of heart disease or stroke may not be a good idea. Undoubtedly, there are other unhealthy foods allowed in The Three Rules plan. I can't cover every food. If you're concerned about food that might be bad for you, don't eat it or eat less. There are countless ways that we can be healthier. For most people, weight is the most significant problem. Stick to The Three Rules, and you will solve that problem. After that, if you want to tackle other health issues related to food, that's up to you, and I recommend it.

Are There Fat-Burning Foods or Foods You Have to Eat to Lose Weight?

You have probably seen claims of a food "burning fat." There is no such thing. Eating any specific food never helps any diet—it's what you remove from your diet, what you no longer eat, that matters. Eating an allowed food does not negate the effects of a prohibited food. Fiber in the diet can blunt glucose rise and help some. Protein and fat in a meal can also lessen the increase in glucose from eating sugar. But eating protein, fat, or fiber doesn't burn fat or cause weight loss.

Many times, as I explained Rule 2 to a patient, they asked what I had eaten for dinner the evening before. I answered sautéed shrimp or chicken and Brussels sprouts. A frequent response was that they didn't like Brussels sprouts. This also happened with yogurt, protein drinks, and even apples. Fine, there are many things I don't like to eat either. Eating Brussels sprouts isn't the important thing. Eating all the vegetables in the world doesn't help. But it doesn't hurt. When you remove the fettuccine alfredo, you have to replace it with something. You are good if you replace it with shrimp and Brussels sprouts, steak and a Caesar salad, or just steak. The important thing is that you do not have pasta and dinner rolls. That is the crux of The Three Rules. Since I have to eat something, I sometimes choose shrimp or chicken and Brussels sprouts, but I could choose from a nearly infinite variety of foods. Nothing you eat will burn fat. It's the removal of junk food that burns the fat. You replace junk food with whatever you want that is within the Three Rules. I am confident you will be able to find some foods you like.

Dried Fruit

The most popular dried fruit is raisins. Grapes have some sugar but are not a problem on The Three Rules. It takes a lot of grapes to raise your sugar, so the glycemic load is reasonably low, and we rarely eat massive amounts of grapes in a sitting. Raisins have the issue of allowing us to eat much more at one time, making it possible to overdo it. But I don't worry about it. No one gets fat on raisins. Raisins do not raise our blood glucose to the level added sugar or other prohibited foods do.

Other commonly encountered dried fruits are prunes, apricots, figs, dates, cranberries, cherries, and mangoes. Like raisins, they usually aren't a problem. If you eat any of these foods to excess, you will probably experience a gastrointestinal disturbance before the sugar becomes a problem. I haven't seen dried fruit interfere with anyone's weight loss. If you ate 5 or 6 servings of dried mango in a sitting, I suppose it could, but I doubt that will be an issue for you. I have mentioned that some foods, such as brown rice, are prohibited because their glycemic load is high enough that you would have to moderate your intake. If you are a dried mango addict, you are probably the only one. I would then consider not eating it at all. Otherwise, no one got fat on dried mangoes.

Remember, I assume you are reading the labels and paying attention to Rule 1. Many dried fruits, especially cranberries, blueberries, cherries, and mangoes, have added sugar. Read every single label of everything you eat. Do you want to ruin your diet plans on dried blueberries because there is added sugar? You could have eaten fresh or frozen blueberries, a fresh mango, an apple, or anything else. Dried fruits are fine. Dried fruits with added sugar are not.

Non-Nutritive Sweeteners

We know that sugar-sweetened food is harmful, causing weight gain, diabetes, and a host of other obesity-related problems. Sugar has also been linked to cancers, heart disease, and other disorders unrelated to weight, and we act as if we're addicted to sugar. But what about non-nutritive (artificial) sweeteners?

Non-nutritive sweeteners have zero sugar, zero carbs, and usually zero or negligible calories. Aspartame (Equal), sucralose (Splenda), and stevia (Truvia and others) are the most popular. Some are natural, others not, but that doesn't necessarily make them good or bad. Tobacco is natural and harmful, and so is sugar.

We consume most of our non-nutritive sweeteners in diet drinks, especially diet sodas, and some people drink quite a bit. When I was in medical school, my roommate and I went through so much Diet Coke that it was embarrassing. Even now, I occasionally binge on diet soda, drinking several a day for weeks. Then I realize what I'm doing and stop for a while. As with many things we like, an occasional treat can become a habit.

Are the sweeteners harmful? For the purposes of weight control, they are fine unless there are other additives. Occasionally, people may develop gastrointestinal symptoms from sucralose or migraines from aspartame. Some experts believe that using artificial sweeteners increases appetite. That may be true, but with The Three Rules, it isn't much of an issue. Recently, there has been a concern about non-nutritive sweeteners and cardiovascular disease. In one study, non-nutritive sweeteners were associated with a slightly increased risk of strokes and heart attacks.[27] Stevia and monk fruit were not consumed enough in the study to draw conclusions about them, and at least two studies show stevia to be safe.[28] [29]

---

[27] Debras C, Chazelas E, Sellem L, et al. Artificial sweeteners and risk of cardiovascular diseases: results from the prospective NutriNet-Santé cohort. BMJ. 2022;378:e071204. Published 2022 Sep 7. doi:10.1136/bmj-2022-071204

[28] Chan P, Tomlinson B, Chen YJ, Liu JC, Hsieh MH, Cheng JT. A double-blind placebo-controlled study of the effectiveness and tolerability of oral stevioside in human hypertension. Br J Clin Pharmacol. 2000;50(3):215-220. doi:10.1046/j.1365-2125.2000.00260.x

[29] Samuel P, Ayoob KT, Magnuson BA, et al. Stevia Leaf to Stevia Sweetener: Exploring Its Science, Benefits, and Future Potential. J Nutr. 2018;148(7):1186S-1205S. doi:10.1093/jn/nxy102

There is another group of low-calorie ingredients called sugar alcohols. They include erythritol, maltitol, xylitol, and other "ols." You'll find them in low-sugar food products such as protein bars and candy. They are not quite zero calories, but we can consider sugar alcohols sugar-free and zero carbs. They are fine on the Three Rules plan, but in excess, all sugar alcohols, except possibly erythritol, can cause diarrhea and bloating. I avoid them because I am susceptible to these side effects, but you are free to try them.

Recently, a study in Nature Medicine suggested that sugar alcohols, especially erythritol, may increase the risk of stroke or heart attack.[30] However, it's possible that some of the erythritol measured was naturally derived from internal processes in the study participants. Rather than consume erythritol, I buy pure stevia for my protein powder (NOW Foods brand), which has no additives.

I told my patients that artificial sweeteners may have risks but nowhere near the problems caused by sugar. If your choice is regular soda or diet soda, drink diet soda. If your choice is diet soda or water, tea, or coffee, drink the water, tea, or coffee. All sugar-free sweeteners are acceptable on the Three Rules plan and should not interfere with losing weight or keeping it off. I try not to use them much because I develop a habit, as I do with many things. And even though they are generally safe, I don't like eating something that isn't definitively good for me, especially if it's hard for me to quit.

---

[30] Witkowski M, Nemet I, Alamri H, et al. The artificial sweetener erythritol and cardiovascular event risk. Nat Med. 2023;29(3):710-718. doi:10.1038/s41591-023-02223-9

A Few More Words About Food Additives

I have said many times that if you are going to break The Rules, then do it with intent and make it count. Nowhere is this more important than food additives. It is a shame to fail in your diet because of a food additive you don't even taste. Sweeteners from the list of about 60 different names for sugar are easy to spot. If you aren't sure, look it up.

In the chapter on Rule 3, we talked about starchy food additives. Some of these have chemical-sounding names, such as maltodextrin. It is added to many mixes and bars, and it's converted to glucose easily. Avoid it altogether (unless you have no other choice and the content is negligible). Various starches are often added to subtly change the taste of food and to thicken it. These are common in low-fat foods, replacing the fat's effect on texture. When the word starch is on the label, don't eat it. You might see corn starch, tapioca starch, or modified food starch.

Thickening sauces within The Rules can be a challenge. You can try various gums, such as guar gum and xanthan gum. If you use them at home, read instructions online because they don't work like flour or corn starch. Be aware that a thickened sauce at a restaurant usually has flour or corn starch.

Carrageenan, made from seaweed, is a food additive making the rounds on the internet. It's put into many beverages, such as soy and almond milk. It has no carbs and no calories and won't affect your diet. You don't taste it, so there is no risk of developing a habit. Some, but not all, studies suggest there may be health risks in consuming it in large amounts for extended periods. For the purposes of The Rules, carrageenan is fine. If you believe the negative stories, avoid it if you want.

There are far too many food additives to name them all. New ones and alternative names for old ones appear regularly. I look them all up. Even with the internet, it can be challenging to determine if a specific additive is against The Rules. As mentioned, the FDA allows a small amount of carbs and calories in sugar-free, zero-calorie products. Be careful unless you know that the product doesn't affect blood sugar and cause weight gain. If it's another name for sugar or starch, don't eat it. The best way to check is to look up the glycemic index. If the index is lower than about 20, it's probably fine. I am not saying the additive is good for you, but it's unlikely to ruin your diet. Do not ruin your diet by eating something you don't even taste. Again, eat with intent. If you go off the Three Rules, make it count.

A Few Other Issues

Not everything is about the actual eating.
You can help yourself in other ways.

We have discussed all you need to know about eating within The Three Rules. All the rest is follow-through. A few things not directly related to eating will help you succeed: exercise, cooking, and shopping.

What About Exercise?

I talked about exercise earlier. It is so important and so often misunderstood that I want to go into more detail. Exercise is unnecessary with The Three Rules, and exercise doesn't prevent weight gain if you don't eat right. Patients told me all the time that they gained twenty or more pounds because something interfered with their activity level or their ability to exercise. It was winter, their job became more sedentary, they had family stress, or they suffered an injury. Lack of exercise is rarely, if ever, the genuine cause of weight gain. Few people gain weight, regardless of activity level or exercise, without eating too much of the wrong food. Fortunately, you can lose weight and keep it off despite not exercising.

Does exercise help with weight loss? Of course, it does, but not much if you don't change your diet. Exercise aids weight loss by burning fat and blunting any rise in glucose in the blood, making fat storage less efficient. Aerobic exercise also helps lower the risk of many medical problems, especially cardiovascular disease. Over the last several years, strength training, such as weightlifting, has been shown to have additional health benefits. Almost everything tested improves with strength training: muscle mass, fat loss, diabetes, cholesterol levels, cardiovascular disease, stroke risk, bone strength, depression, and even overall mortality. Low muscle strength is an independent predictor of premature death, as seen in this study and many others.[31] I recommend that nearly everyone engage in aerobic and strength training.

For overall health, I exercise aerobically nearly every day and add strength training three days a week. Since I follow The Rules, I don't need to exercise to keep my weight down—I work out for all the other benefits. I have to eat more when I exercise to avoid losing too much weight. And when I burn more calories than usual, like on a hiking trip to Glacier National Park, I have to eat much more, or I come home several pounds low. I usually eat more dried fruit, whole grains, and nuts when exercising that much. Remember, gaining weight on The Rules is not impossible, but it is difficult. But that doesn't mean you will gain weight just because you don't exercise. Just stay strict with The Rules.

---

[31] Ortega FB, Silventoinen K, Tynelius P, Rasmussen F. Muscular strength in male adolescents and premature death: cohort study of one million participants. BMJ. 2012;345:e7279. Published 2012 Nov 20. doi:10.1136/bmj.e7279

I recommend you exercise. Do it every day, if possible, but at least 3-4 days per week. It helps with overall health and weight management, but more importantly, it helps you make the right food choices. When we exercise, we feel better physically and about ourselves. We have a sense of accomplishment, leading to good, healthy choices. After 45 minutes on a treadmill or lifting weights, I wouldn't consider eating junk food and ruining it. Skipping planned exercise, for whatever reason, can lead to the attitude, "Screw it. I didn't exercise; I might as well give up on the entire day and eat at McDonald's." I've done it myself too many times to count.

When patients attributed their twenty-pound weight gain to their lack of exercise, there are two points I tried to mention tactfully. First, you don't gain twenty pounds by lack of exercise alone. It takes a change in eating habits. Some people honestly believe that their diet hasn't changed. But it can be subtle: a few more restaurant meals or takeout, an extra dessert at night, two more beers in the evening. If you eat right, on The Three Rules, you won't gain weight, whether or not you exercise.

The other point I make is more important. You can almost always find a way to exercise and stay active, regardless of what happens in your life. Of course, a true family crisis takes precedence over exercise. Otherwise, you can usually find time to walk outside, go up and down stairs at the library, march in place for twenty minutes watching television, walk in the mall if the weather is bad, or go to the gym. Even a broken leg will not stop you if you're motivated. You can do upper body exercise with push-ups against the sofa, lift light weights over and over, or, if allowed, walk with crutches—which is far more exercise than walking without a broken leg. It's difficult exercising with an injury or marching in place for twenty minutes when the weather is terrible outside, but who said life was easy? At the beginning of the book, I said losing weight is hard. Exercise is hard, too. Do it anyway.

How To Cook

Obviously, there is no way I can teach you to cook in a book like this. I cook most days, but it would be a stretch to say I'm talented. Fortunately, you don't need to be a chef to make healthy, tasty meals that follow The Three Rules. You shouldn't need any advice on preparing most breakfasts and lunches. You can manage scrambled eggs, yogurt and fruit, a cheese plate, vegetables and peanut butter, and tuna salad.

What about dinner, the meal most of us look forward to? I divide dinners into two categories: casual and formal. Most weekday meals are casual. A more formal meal would be on the weekends, and a truly formal dinner would be for parties or holidays.

What I am writing here only applies to a few of you because you likely have more cooking skills and a better imagination than I do. If you skip the rest of this section, I promise I'm okay with it. Most casual meals I make center on protein, like steak, chicken, fish, or beans. A side of vegetables or a salad would be typical. Look for recipes online or in books on how to prepare them the way you like them. Many websites let you search "low carb." I assume you know the sites or can find them, but I use the free sites SeriousEats.com, FoodNetwork.com, Food.com, and Allrecipes.com the most. For a subscription, AmericasTestKitchen.com.com is superb, and I've learned most of my favorite recipes from them. Many low-carb recipes online do not wholly adhere to The Three Rules. That's fine since it is simple, with a few tweaks, to make the meal fit The Rules. If there is added sugar, use sucralose, stevia, or aspartame, calculating the amount based on the recommendations on the sweeteners' labels. If there is a thickener such as corn starch or flour, leave it unthickened, or thicken it with xanthan gum, guar gum, flaxseed, or a few other products you can find online. As I said, read the instructions since I have ruined a dish or two with some of these thickeners. You can also use puréed lentils or mung beans to thicken a soup.

A formal meal requires more attention and practice because I want to ensure everything runs smoothly. I spend extra time making it perfect, and if I've altered the recipe significantly, I try it out before serving it to others. When we have a big party with multiple courses, we may make some dishes that are against The Rules. I don't eat it, just as some vegans serve meat to guests and do not eat it themselves. Don't make the sweet potato casserole for Thanksgiving if you think it will tempt you. Some people have no trouble eating whatever they want during a holiday, returning to their diet plan the next day. I can't always do that, so I don't eat food against The Rules at formal meals. There is always more than enough to eat at a holiday dinner that is within The Rules.

Many of you may have a family member who is not on your diet plan. When home from college, our son often ate junk food and bad carbs. That was up to him, but he ate dinner with us and ate what we did. Sometimes, if he had a friend over, we'd make a separate side dish, like a rice pilaf—I know I can always avoid eating rice. When our son was young, I sometimes made a separate meal for him. It was more work, but it was worth it for me not to eat the spaghetti marinara he wanted for dinner.

Ideally, everyone in your household would eat as you want to eat, but I know that isn't always practical. I frequently hear from someone who blames their failure at a diet on their spouse, who is an outstanding cook and makes food that is against The Rules—they might make the best bread or homemade cinnamon buns. You will have to decide how important your weight is to you. I believe it is the most critical health concern for non-smokers. So, I do what I think is best, regardless. You can always tell the baker in the family that you appreciate it but don't want to eat it. My alcohol analogy applies here as well. I often received gifts of wine from patients who were connoisseurs, and I politely told them I didn't drink. I am sure vegans do the same when their loved ones want to make them a prime rib for their birthday.

How To Shop

Most foods are healthy and good for our weight, but we tend to eat the few bad ones. After describing The Three Rules, I am frequently asked, "What do you eat?" A better question is, "What do you buy?" There are free samples at stores, dinners at a friend's house, and treats people bring to the office, but we purchase most of what we eat—at a grocery store, restaurant, or gas station.

When buying the food yourself, controlling what you eat is easier. You have two steps to avoid breaking a Rule: don't buy it, and then don't eat it. We all know that you're likely to eat it once you purchase it, even if you tell yourself it's for a special occasion or for your child or spouse. If it's in the house, you must always have willpower. This is why someone who wants to quit smoking should never keep cigarettes in the house and why people with an alcohol problem shouldn't keep alcohol in the home. If temptation is right in front of you for hours a day, you must have discipline for hours each day. I rarely keep bad carbs in the house, so I only need willpower at the store. The rare times I have junk food in the house—like when my wife and son make Christmas treats—I have to be careful. I try never to have junk food at home, and I never buy it.

What do you do if you live with others who don't want to stick to The Three Rules? You have a few options. Ideally, you would convince them of the value of The Rules. This works best if you have a spouse or partner with a weight issue. Then, you both should avoid keeping bad carbs at home. If you have a child, you are the boss and can make your own rules. If none of that is feasible, then you may have to buy the food they want. Once they have followed The Three Rules for a while, some people can see bad carbs around the house and not eat them. For most people, me included, it's too difficult to avoid eating junk food that's constantly around them. You can make a deal with your spouse, child, or roommate. Have an area of the pantry or refrigerator that is off-limits to you. You can even lock it up. Putting a lock on a drawer or cabinet isn't difficult. It seems drastic, but if it helps you conquer your weight problem, do it. Some parents lock their liquor cabinets, so locking a junk food cabinet is not unprecedented.

Do not cave in and buy junk food at the store on a whim. The best prevention is a list—always go in with a list. That gives you a failsafe to keep you following The Rules: Do not put junk food on the list, and don't buy anything not on the list. Then you will not have it in the house and won't eat it. Easy.

At the store, you will spend most of your time in the produce, meat, seafood, and dairy sections. You may stop at a few other aisles to get frozen fruit or vegetables, condiments, and kitchen staples. Stay away from the bakery, prepared foods section, cereal aisle, or candy aisle. Avoid snacks unless you have nuts on your list. (I believe the best place to buy nuts is Costco—the highest quality and lowest prices.) Stay away from the parts of the store with foods that are against The Rules. Be careful at the ends of the aisles and at checkout, where they sell especially tempting junk food.

Before buying food that has a label, read the ingredients. Repeating myself, it isn't grams of carbs or grams of sugar in the section called "Nutrition Facts" that is important. I look at this area because they often write about added sugars, which should be zero. They also list protein and fiber in the nutrition area. But it's the added sugar, which is always listed in the ingredients, that matters—remember that there are multiple names for sugars and refined carbs. I know I ceaselessly mention reading the label. It is critically important. Don't buy anything without reading the label.

Part 5

Keeping It Off Forever

*Losing weight and gaining it back is demoralizing.
Don't let it happen.*

would be surprised if you've never lost weight and regained it. I have already told you how I've done it repeatedly. You may have heard of studies showing how this "yo-yo" of weight has health risks. That isn't the biggest problem. It's demoralizing. We regret the weight gain and call ourselves stupid and weak. Feeling ashamed can then lead to more unhealthy choices. It can make it more difficult to start another diet because we think we will only regain the weight. If you look back to when the weight started returning, it's usually after a few days of poor food choices and lack of attention. It is rarely, if ever, that we say, "I want to just eat what I want, and I don't care if I regain the weight."

The Three Rules to Lose Weight and Keep It Off Forever is just what it says. The Rules work forever. There is not much difference between the Rules plan when you are losing weight and keeping it off—in fact, you eat the same way. There is no transition from losing weight to keeping it off. I told patients starting on The Three Rules that they did not need a target weight or a goal amount to lose. You will lose the excess weight and stay there.

For most people, there is nothing more to do once you lose the weight—keep following The Rules. A few people will begin to lose too much weight. This uncommon problem is easily managed, and we will discuss it. Generally, to keep the weight off, keep doing what you're doing, and your weight will remain stable.

As this part of the book will describe, staying focused is the main difficulty in keeping weight off. For the rest of your life, you will be tempted to break The Rules. Intentionally or not, people will encourage you to break them. You will have good days and challenging days, and you will consider returning to old habits. I will go over some ways to avoid slipping. Remember what I have said—losing weight is hard. Keeping weight off forever may be more challenging. Do it anyway.

Losing Weight Vs. Keeping It Off

When you follow the Three Rules, you will lose excess fat. You will naturally stay at the new weight.

Until the recent boom in the wealth and security of the Western world, we mainly ate within the Three Rules. We ate little sugar or refined carbs, and when we ate starchy vegetables, it wasn't in today's quantities. Junk food was difficult to find. There was no fast food, takeout, pizza delivery, etc. When we ate bad carbs, the amount of exercise we did overwhelmed it. So, we rarely needed to lose weight, and when we did, our work and diet kept us from gaining it back. Fortunately, even in our modern lives, we will stay at a healthy weight if we continue to follow The Rules.

Should I Change the Rules?

You or someone you care about wants to and needs to lose weight. Start following The Three Rules right now. If you follow through on this commitment, you are set for life. Just follow through. There are unique challenges when you have lost the excess weight (fat, not muscle) and are trying to keep it off. In theory, it's simple. Keep doing what you were doing. Follow The Rules. There are times, though, when you may want to or need to change The Rules. Do it with intent.

Why would you want to change The Rules when you are doing well? You shouldn't consider a significant change, such as eating bad carbs in moderation, because the risk of relapse is too high. There are only two times to consider modifying The Rules, even in a small way. The first reason is risky: you may want to try a prohibited food again. The second is if you are losing too much weight. This is uncommon, and I will deal with it soon.

I do not recommend trying a prohibited food just because you miss eating it. I never do it myself because I know I will be unable to stop. You may not be quite as addicted as I am, so you may consider making a minor change. You may allow corn, sweet potatoes, or white rice—all prohibited by Rule 3. You might be tempted to try eating one candy bar a week. Again, this is risky. If you do it, start very small and don't give up the benefit of having a strict Rule to follow, so make a Rule Variation, as we discussed with brown rice. Say to yourself that Rule 3 is now, "Do not eat starchy vegetables or fruits, except rice or sweet potatoes, or whatever." If you risk a candy bar a week, change Rule 1 to "Don't eat any food with added sugar except one Snickers bar on Sunday." That way, there is a strict Rule again, and you can be accountable. Vague rules inevitably lead to failure. Don't wing it by saying that you partly obey Rule 3. Make your own new Rule 3 with the Variation. If you try something so risky, I strongly urge you to weigh yourself every few days. If you gain weight, return to the absolute strictest you can be with the Three Rules, without the Variation.

There are many other Variations of The Rules that my readers have created. Some add one processed and refined carbohydrate food weekly or even daily, while others add pizza twice a month. A few people succeed, but most fail, allowing more and more prohibited food to creep back into their diet. It's up to you, but please be careful. The foods you add back are usually not worth the downside of gaining your weight back. I cannot stress enough that if you tweak a Rule, keep a strict Rule with a Variation, with wording that includes your added foods.

Focus Every Day

We do many positive things every day, even when we are unhealthy in others. Most of us brush our teeth, shower, kiss our loved ones, and tuck our kids into bed, yet attention to our diet is somehow not worth doing every day. We rate our health as one of our top priorities but don't act that way, and unless you smoke, what you eat is the most important thing for your health.

If you follow The Rules, you will succeed. Do it every day. Focus every day. Focusing on my diet helps me focus on everything else in my life. In the past, when I lost focus and gained weight back, I also lost focus on other important things. I stopped exercising, drank more alcohol, or mindlessly flipped channels on television. We should have leisure time—relaxation, vacations, and so on. But think about it—do you stop brushing your teeth and showering on a vacation? Do you suddenly start doing drugs on a cruise? If you want to succeed in anything, you have to focus. This is especially true with habit-forming things like bad carbs.

We lose focus on our diet for many reasons—injury, illness, job stress, holidays, a busy time, and occasionally serious crises.

Sometimes, we allow a friend to talk us into eating an addicting snack or dessert. We may feel bad saying no to office colleagues bearing treats. Whatever it is, we all are prone to losing concentration and diverting our attention from something important, like our health. We are imperfect, so don't waste energy on guilt or self-recrimination. If you lose focus, and it will likely happen, recognize it and start immediately again with The Rules. If you slip up with any important goal in life, don't wait. Don't put it off until the following day or week. Regain focus immediately, the same day, or even the moment you lose it.

What If I Lose Too Much?

It may seem difficult to believe, but The Rules are so effective that some people continue to lose weight after they reach their goal. Sometimes, they had set their target weight too high, not realizing that with The Three Rules, their weight would continue to come off. Occasionally, the target weight is reasonable, and they continue to lose weight, becoming too thin. This has happened to me. You may think it's a good problem to have, and I would rather lose too much weight (without illness) than gain too much weight. There are risks, however. In this situation, it's tempting to start eating bad carbs like potatoes in one meal and a dessert in the next. Just like a cheat day or going off The Rules when you have a bad day or are too busy to cook, it often leads quickly to regaining weight.

If you lose too much weight, I recommend two things. First, find something within The Rules you like; in my case, it's nuts. I roast raw almonds and walnuts and usually eat a cup and a half a day, about a thousand calories. Since I'm 5 foot 5 inches, that's a lot of calories, given that I also eat three meals daily. It usually keeps my weight steady. Adding a lot of whole grains such as barley or quinoa can also stop unwanted weight loss.

If you prefer fruit to nuts, fine; eat much more fruit than you were eating while losing weight. Bananas, being a borderline fruit, would be an excellent choice, as would grapes—fine overall in The Rules but relatively high in sugar. Eating vast quantities of grapes might overwhelm your system and cause some weight gain or at least minimize unwanted weight loss. You could also eat two portions of whatever protein you serve for dinner, extra servings of vegetables, or more cheese. If you eat an enormous amount of anything, even within The Rules, you will likely stop losing weight. I mentioned earlier that it is possible to fail to lose weight or even to gain weight within The Rules, but it's difficult. The Three Rules will not necessarily work if you do something crazy or ridiculous. If you do what I recommended, while not crazy or ridiculous, it should stop you from losing too much weight. Monitor your weight, and when you stop losing, go back to what you were doing before. It should be easy to cut back on the foods you just added unless you added something addictive, like ice cream.

This will almost always stop your weight loss, but if you continue to lose weight or cannot eat more of any foods within The Rules, you can try adding something against The Rules, but please create a Rule Variation. Use something not typically as habit-forming as sugar—like rice, corn, or sweet potato. I don't recommend you eat potatoes. The same holds for candy, pastries, or bread rolls. They are all just too addictive, and like a cheat day, you are risking regaining all your weight back.

Whatever you do, I strongly recommend naming it a Rule Variation. That way, you maintain the benefit of All or None. You still follow The Rules; you just tweak one of them. Then, you can say to yourself for Rule 3, "Do not eat starchy vegetables or fruit—but I will eat sweet potatoes every other day." Or "Do not eat any food with processed…except oatmeal three days a week." You get the idea. Make a Rule Variation and stick to it.

I generally recommend not weighing yourself often. However, if you make a Rule Variation, weigh yourself at least weekly. When you stop losing weight, back off on what you added to your diet. If you see a continued weight gain trend, eliminate the Variation and return to the strict Rules. I don't have an exact recommendation on the amount of weight gain, but I would not wait long. If you've lost a few pounds more than you think you should have, stop the Variation when you gain that back. You may have to try different Variations in different amounts until you find the right balance.

I wouldn't spend too much time on this issue since it isn't typical. In most people, sticking to The Rules is all you need to do. You're not likely to lose more than you want. If it happens, if you pay close attention to what you are doing, there is little risk in making a minor Variation to The Rules. But don't lose focus. If you make a tweak and you don't weigh yourself, you're likely to put it out of your mind. You may regain your weight and be right back where you started. I have seen it many times.

Part 6

Tips and Traps or How to Live on The Three Rules

Here is a grab bag of lessons I have learned over the years. Most of these pearls of wisdom came from my own mistakes and failures. I have already mentioned some tips in various parts of the book, but I hope you will at least briefly read and think about them again. To work this hard and fail because of something avoidable is frustrating. We all make plenty of mistakes. Learning from someone else's is nice once in a while.

I couldn't group each tip or pitfall in a perfectly sensible way, and I will simply go from one to the next. Many will be more important later in your plan when you have lost the weight and are keeping it off, but it can help to at least read about them now so you can be ready for everything.

All Or None

For the last time, I promise, All or None is critically important if your end in mind is losing all your excess weight. You are either following The Three Rules, or you are not. I know you will succeed if you are All In and may fail if you are not All In. Most experts believe this is the best approach for any addiction or recurring problem, such as alcohol, drugs, or gambling. Bad carbs, especially sugars, are similar. An alcoholic cannot get into trouble with alcohol if they don't have the first drink. No one can get into trouble with Oreos if they don't have the first bite.

Changing The Rules

You may be tempted to go off The Rules, in a small way with one of the Variations I mentioned, or dramatically with multiple cheat days each week. It's your choice, but I have one recommendation if you do—wait until you first master The Three Rules. Like any new endeavor, you want to succeed with strict rules before making changes. When we had new staff in our office, we wanted to ensure they knew how to do things correctly first. Then, they could fine-tune their work, cutting a small corner or two, and still be successful. If you bend The Rules from the start and fail, you cannot determine the cause of the failure. I strongly recommend you follow The Rules to the letter. Then, after you have success, if you feel the need to bend a Rule, start with small steps. Make a Rule Variation and pay close attention to your weight so you can return to The Rules strictly if your weight goes up. You will immediately be back on track and lose weight again right away.

Eat With Intent

Every time you get ready to eat something, consider whether you want to eat it. Eat with intent. We are better off if we always act with intent. There would be far fewer accidents, fights, and obesity if we did. Just thinking, "Do I want to eat this?" usually keeps us from eating it.

If you decide to break a Rule, do it with intent. You are less likely to regret it, and regret leads to further failures. If you mindlessly eat a bag of powdered donuts, you will regret it. If you feel it is the right thing to eat a Krispy Kreme chocolate glazed, then do it, do it with intent, and go right back to The Rules. Then you will succeed. You will lose weight, just not that day.

Make Your Own Meals

Make your own meals. I know I'm repeating myself, but it's important for The Three Rules, health in general, and many other reasons. When you buy and prepare the food, you will know that everything you eat and drink is within The Rules. You have infinite options, so there is no excuse for eating bad carbs if you make the food. It's that simple.

The idea that healthy food is expensive is simply not true. Chicken, fish, beef, pork, and shellfish are all reasonably priced. I mention Costco's prices because that's where I shop, but low prices are available at many stores. Two whole chickens for fourteen dollars, salmon at $9.99 a pound, various cuts of meat at $3.99 a pound, and so on. I bought a 5-pound leg of lamb for $5.99 a pound and an excellent bone-in ham for $2.99 a pound for Christmas dinner. It served ten of us, and we had a ton and a half for leftovers. I also made a bean dish—it was nearly free. The biggest meal of the year, for ten people, with leftovers, was about $60. The average dinner at my house is well under $10, and many are under $5.

Books have been written on the value of sitting down to a family dinner. The more we eat and socialize with our loved ones, the better. Takeout and restaurants rarely lead to meaningful conversations that strengthen relationships.

Preparing a meal is only a chore if you decide it's a chore. I plan meals for the week and usually shop just once. Most weekday meals are simple, but I make more elaborate dinners on weekends. Sometimes they are not so good. So what? That's how we learn. Cooking gives you a sense of accomplishment and can be a joy in and of itself. My wife just made pajamas for our son. I know many people who knit for fun, giving gifts to grandchildren or charity. Knitting and sewing may have been considered chores at one time, but now they are hobbies. Cooking is the same thing, though I'm the first to admit that my usual meal isn't in the same league as my son's pajamas or the multi-colored scarf I received from a patient. Embrace cooking as a fun, relaxing activity that saves money and helps you become healthy.

Do Not Keep Junk Food at Home

If you are at a restaurant, you must have willpower for about an hour to avoid bad carbs. If you go into a gas station, you must be disciplined for a few minutes. If you're at home, and there is junk food, you must be perfect continuously. Anything can slip you up.

You're hungry and see the Oreo cookies. There's a problem at work, so you get home and want a Dove chocolate bar. You allow yourself one bagel because your sister is staying with you. There is no limit to our excuses, allowing ourselves to stray from our plan. If the food is not in your home, you will not eat it in the home. It's that simple. Why set yourself up for failure? If a reformed alcoholic keeps alcohol in their home, their risk of relapse is high.

We live in the actual world. Many of us live with others, and they may not have the same ideas as you. They may want to keep bad carbs in the house. This can be managed, but it takes some work. The options are simple:

- You can insist that the food not be in the home. This requires a frank discussion, and depending on the relationship, it may be impossible.
- You can make them keep the food in an area you don't use, like a closet or small refrigerator.
- You can put bad carbs under lock and key.

Don't keep bad carbs in the home until following The Rules becomes a habit, and you can avoid eating junk food even if it's within reach. I had to do it 100% when I started. Now, I can make exceptions, mainly during the holidays when my wife makes treats. I can now look at a homemade caramel and not eat one or ten.

These measures seem drastic, but being obese requires drastic measures. People with asthma don't allow smoking in the house, those with newborns don't let sick people visit, and pregnant women do not drink alcohol at all. Overweight people with an addiction to bad carbs don't allow junk food in the home.

Fat-Burning Foods and Required Foods (Again)

We discussed this before, and it's worth repeating. There are no foods you can eat that will cause weight loss. A few foods may help you lose weight indirectly. Eggs and other proteins eaten early in the day may suppress appetite later. Cinnamon and some high-fiber foods may lower the glycemic index in a meal. But there are no foods that cause weight loss themselves. The key to The Three Rules is removing bad carbs (junk food) from your diet. Remove it entirely. Then, replace what you give up with any food you want that follows The Rules. Steak and green beans do not burn fat; giving up the hamburger bun and fries does.

Do not eat junk food. Eat what's in The Rules. Try to ignore what you read and hear about fat-burning foods. Do not pay attention to get-thin-quick supplements or schemes. Even if they work, and they usually don't, you won't keep the weight off. You will learn nothing from it, and you will not have the sense of accomplishment from doing something yourself.

The Goal Should Be Absolute Adherence to The Rules.

I cannot stress this enough. The Rules work if you stick to them. All or None works. Less than All or None may not and usually does not work. Do not expect this to be simple all the time. Every failure of The Rules plan or other diets occurs when there is not strict adherence. In a low-calorie diet, you will probably fail if you have a few hundred extra calories here or there. If you are on Weight Watchers, eat a few extra points, and you will fail. I ask patients what they are doing to lose weight, and they often say, "I'm kind of doing South Beach" or "Sort of counting calories." They are rarely successful.

Lack of strict adherence to The Three Rules is the same. But since there are only Three Rules and so many delicious foods within The Rules, it can be done. It is hard. Do it anyway.

Mind Tricks and Mantras

I have mentioned many techniques that have helped me and my patients stick to The Rules. You can think of junk food (bad carbs) as a dangerous drug or addictive activity to help you avoid eating a treat at work. You can think of cheating on The Rules as cheating on a spouse. I often call them mind tricks, but trick may not be the right word. They are motivational techniques to accomplish the task at hand.

Another technique is to think only of today as if today is all there is. Remember that the present is all we know for sure that we have. When working on a diet plan or any positive change in your life, it's daunting if you think in terms of years, months, or even days. Patients sometimes asked me, "Do I need to do this forever?" First, you don't need to do anything; you can live with your weight problem. But I said, "No, you just don't eat junk food today." You only follow The Rules today. When tomorrow comes, you do the same thing. All we have is today, so eat healthy today. This is the opposite of what we usually do when eating junk food. We say we will only eat it today and then keep eating it for days. What I want you to accomplish is to eat well today. Tomorrow, another day, you do the same thing.

Any mental technique or mind trick you can use is good. You will know what works for you. I use mantras—words or statements you repeat for motivation, relaxation, or self-improvement. I use a few to help me relax in tough situations and to motivate myself to accomplish difficult tasks. When especially challenged, I use the phrase "The Obstacle Is the Way" from the book I mentioned. Another favorite is "It is hard, do it anyway." When everyone is eating bagels and lox, you might see me mouthing, "Do it anyway."

None of these techniques are magic. They won't cure a serious addiction and may not make you a concert pianist, but mind tricks and mantras can get you through a moment of weakness. When a tray of cookies is passed your way, picturing heroin syringes may help you say, "No, thanks." When at a restaurant, repeating a mantra may help you order the Caesar salad with chicken rather than the burger and fries.

Find Foods You Like

This is the fun part. When you start any diet or healthy lifestyle, you must give something up. If you cut calories, you give up some high-calorie foods you enjoy. On The Three Rules, you give up foods with bad carbs. Since these foods make up much of the American diet, and you have a weight problem, you probably eat junk food daily. It can be challenging to think of what you will eat in the future. As I mentioned, I am frequently asked, "So, what do you eat?"

Fortunately, although Americans eat a lot of junk food, it makes up a tiny percentage of our food options.

I suggest you go to a standard grocery store today. You don't need to go to a fancy boutique store or Whole Foods, though that is fine, too. Just walk up and down every aisle and look around. Most of the produce area is within The Rules, and many fruits and vegetables may be unknown to you. Write down things to look up later or look them up right away on a smartphone. (I've been doing this for a while and still need to look up some fruits and vegetables.)

Most grocery stores have a standard and specialty cheese section. (Costco is the least expensive, as always), and I predict there are at least twenty cheeses you have never tried. The entire meat and seafood section, excluding a few prepared foods, is perfect for you. Learn about anything you're not familiar with. Avoid the aisles I mentioned before. The refrigerators have many excellent choices, some prepared, some not. You'll find pickles, sauerkraut (read the label), tofu, yogurt, and other healthy items here. Write down anything you haven't tried before and read about them.

It's often said we should avoid the center aisles of the store, but the Asian and international aisles usually have some excellent choices, and you should definitely check out the spices. Canned fruit generally has added sugar, but there may be canned vegetables and fish you'll like.

Hopefully, walking through the grocery store, you'll find dozens of foods you haven't thought of eating in a while or have never heard of. I recently created a website and plan to post recipes and other tips—haroldoster.com. You can also search for "low carbohydrate recipes" and "keto diet recipes" for ideas. Watch a cooking show. Most recipes can be modified to follow The Rules.

Don't be afraid to experiment. I have no cooking training besides what I learned from my mother-in-law, my wife, books, and the internet. I can only remember one meal I have ever made that was impossible to eat. (Without reading any instructions, I made a sauce thickened with psyllium. It had the consistency of mucus, so we threw the dinner out.)

Create a file or computer database of recipes you like and make them often. You will discover that you can vary the recipes on your own. Most meat recipes will work with chicken, fish, steak, or pork with a few changes. Variations in spices will give you even more options. Will you be able to appear on a food television show? I doubt it, but you will enjoy food, accomplish something on your own, and lose weight.

The key to any lifestyle change or diet is to enjoy it—you'll quit if you don't. I promise you can enjoy eating. I promise there are foods out there that are good. I cannot imagine you not liking at least three dishes we served last Christmas. As we learned as kids, you sometimes have to try things a few times before you can say you genuinely like or dislike them. It took me a couple of times to love hummus and guacamole. Roasted Brussels sprouts were not even on my radar before I changed to a healthy diet. I never thought of roasting bell peppers or zucchini in the oven. Prepared correctly, with the right sauces and spices, these foods are excellent. If you don't make food at home, it's more difficult, but most restaurants have menu items on the Three Rules and will usually make modifications to accommodate you.

I enjoy eating. You will enjoy eating on The Three Rules more than you do now because you'll know it's good for you and that you're accomplishing your goals. Right now is the hard part because you're just starting. You will lose weight and enjoy eating, and it will come automatically in less time than you can imagine.

Restaurants

Restaurants and takeout establishments make it more difficult to follow any diet, including The Three Rules. We discussed the basics. Order foods that follow The Rules, taking care to ask what is in everything you eat. Planning is essential, and I look at the menu online before I go anywhere to eat. If there is absolutely nothing on the menu, then I don't go there. If I must go, I eat at home before or after the meal. However, there are few restaurants where you can't find an entrée or an appetizer, salad, or soup that isn't against The Rules. Don't worry about upsetting the waitstaff. Just order what you want. If there is one side dish within The Rules, order it. Get two if you like, or ask to make it into an entrée. Most people would eat the burger and fries and comfort themselves that there was nothing to eat on the menu. There may not be, but that doesn't mean you have to eat against your plan. Why ruin your diet because of it?

There are many restaurants to choose from. Don't hide your weight loss plan from your friends and family. If they ask if you want to go to a pizza place, say, "No." Many restaurants have choices for you and will also have pizza for them. Find a restaurant that has what you want. More often than not, your friends and family will also find what they want.

Enjoy Eating

Most people who habitually eat junk food don't enjoy eating. We get so used to eating it that we don't enjoy it. Then, we feel guilty, leading to the spiral of weight gain. I saw patients who admitted eating fast food every day. I could easily see they were unhappy about it, and it embarrassed them to admit it. I would bet that if they ate healthily and had a Big Mac and fries every few weeks, they would enjoy that meal much more. You likely won't do well in the long run if you eat fast food occasionally because of the All or None issue, but at least you would be better off than if you were eating it every day.

We should try to enjoy every meal. A well-prepared simple chicken dinner with roasted vegetables is tasty. You don't need fancy foods or a high-priced restaurant to make eating fun. We are not talking about stale bread and gruel. If you don't think about what you eat and grab the easy takeout, you miss out on enjoying healthy, well-prepared meals. When eating with intent, eating healthy, and thinking about meal preparation, you will love eating much more than you did in the past when you were eating bad carbs every day.

Plateaus Or Regaining

After initial success, you may reach a plateau and stop losing weight. You might even gain weight, but that is more common months into the diet. In nearly every case I have seen, in myself and others, it's caused by eating some things against The Rules. It is occasionally obvious, like eating a bagel a few days a week or a cookie at bedtime. But sometimes, it's subtle. The most common culprits are restaurants where the ingredients are unknown and sauces, dressings, and snack foods with processed carbs.

If you plateau or gain weight, I recommend you examine everything you eat or drink. (You should do this anyway, but double your efforts if you're not losing weight.) Write down everything you eat and either confirm the ingredients on the label or search for the ingredient list online. If nothing is against The Rules, look closely at the fruits and vegetables. If there are any possibly starchy ones, stop eating them. If you are drinking smoothies and are not absolutely sure of the ingredients—no additives, no added sugar—stop them.

I have yet to see a single failure where 100% of all food and drink consumed was within The Rules. If you have written everything down for two weeks and are confident that nothing you ate or drank is against The Rules, please get me a message. I would like to record the first example where I have seen The Three Rules break down.

Parties and Other People's Homes

When you are at someone else's home for a party, take the same care you do at a restaurant, though it's easier. There are usually many choices, and no one notices or cares what you eat. You can easily find enough food within The Rules. If you're not sure, ask. That may make you uncomfortable at first, but think of it this way. Every host wants you to be happy and comfortable with the food you eat. When the host is a close friend or family member, they probably already know about your Rules. This is another reason I recommend being open with your loved ones regarding your plans. My family knows I don't eat bad carbs, and I don't drink alcohol. They have a few excellent food choices and don't offer me an alcoholic drink.

A helpful idea is to think like a vegan. A vegan has no trouble asking the host of a party or a restaurant's waitstaff what is in everything served. You can point out your preferences similarly and won't offend anyone. Many medical conditions require a change in diet—allergy, diabetes, hypertension, heart disease, and alcohol dependence. If you add obesity to that list, then we should feel comfortable asking anyone what is in the food we are offered.

Gifts

We all receive gifts of food. It was common for me to get wine, candy, cookies, and other treats each Christmas, though as more patients learned about The Rules, I received fewer and fewer such gifts. I always thanked my patients who were so generous, and if I knew them well, I told them about my habits and how my family or office staff would love the treats. Like hosts at a party, everyone who gives a gift wants the recipient to be happy. When people realize I won't be eating the cookies, there may be a brief period of awkwardness, but I prefer telling them the truth.

One benefit of receiving a gift that I won't eat is that I can give it away. I use a technique recommended in *Don't Sweat the Small Stuff* by Richard Carlson. At work, I gave the treat to someone else and didn't tell anyone, not even the recipient. I left it on their desk with an unsigned note. Everyone was happy.

Office Treats

You can avoid office treats like junk food at parties and bad-carb gifts. Don't have a single bite. The most important first step is to avoid even seeing them. During the holiday season, the treats may be kept in a break room. Don't go in there; it's like not keeping junk food in the home. If you're tempted to eat the office treats, think about whether you would use heroin, smoke cigarettes, or do other harmful things just because they were free and available. Junk food isn't immediately risky, like drugs, but it will ruin your plans and damage your health in the long run. If it helps to think of heroin or cigarettes when you see an office treat, then do it. It is hard to avoid eating treats. Do it anyway.

Travel

Travel is a challenge. Most people eat out nearly every meal on vacation. We discussed how to handle restaurants, but it is never as easy as eating at home. Consider staying at vacation rentals where you have a kitchen and can make anything you want. I find it fun to make dinner with family and friends on vacation. Remember, cooking is only a chore if you decide that it is. You'll also save hundreds of dollars if you avoid even a few restaurant meals on a ten-day trip.

A common theme in this book and something I talk about daily is licensing. We license ourselves to eat junk food on vacation, during holidays, when having an unpleasant day, and when celebrating something. It makes little sense, however.

We can always find a reason to eat junk food, and vacations ruin many diets. Yet, on vacation, we don't smoke, do drugs, or cheat on our spouses. Many people laugh when I say this, but I'm serious. Why is it different? We don't cheat on our spouse or do drugs on vacation because we believe we should never cheat on our spouse or do drugs. However, we think our eating habits are flexible. Many people die each year from obesity and bad eating habits, and I treat my diet as an essential part of my life and well-being. Don't cheat yourself just because you are on vacation.

Holidays

Holidays are a significant stumbling block for many people trying to control their weight. The holiday season starts with Thanksgiving and continues through New Year's Day and beyond. A study in a major medical journal showed that the average person gains just under a pound during the holiday season, and 20% of people gain between two and four pounds.[32] That small amount will add up over the years, but that isn't the biggest problem. The holiday season derails diets. We may have had a few months of healthy eating, but we hit November, and that's the end of it. We have a treat or two, then cookies, candy, pie, and everything else.

This is where everything we just talked about becomes even more important. The All or None approach works for everyone. If you never have the first peanut butter blossom cookie, you can never have

[32] Yanovski JA, Yanovski SZ, Sovik KN, Nguyen TT, O'Neil PM, Sebring NG. A prospective study of holiday weight gain. N Engl J Med. 2000;342(12):861-867. doi:10.1056/NEJM200003233421206

the second. It's hard saying no to the first one. Do it anyway. It is nearly impossible for most of us to say no to the second. Ideally, you would never be around these beautiful treats, and it's one of the few times of the year when I have bad carbs in the house. My wife made blossom cookies, toffee, and chocolate-butterscotch haystacks this year. I know myself. I couldn't have one, or I would have mindlessly gorged on all of them. It was hard.

If you want to lose weight, keep it off, and be healthy, do not have the first holiday treat. If you can see the goodies in your home and abstain, that would be fantastic. In the past, I couldn't do it. Do not be afraid to put up measures to avoid seeing the treats. Don't keep the food in the home, or find a way not to see it.

Cheat Days

You may think my editor made a mistake, with two book sections about cheat days. This redundant passage is intentional since I feel so strongly about it. As you know, a cheat day is a day you allow yourself to "cheat" on a diet. If you're on a low-calorie diet, you could pig out for one day every week. If you're on a carbohydrate-based diet, you could eat fettuccine alfredo or Twix Bars. I don't recommend a cheat day. As I said earlier, I don't like the word "cheat." It implies you are somehow cheating the diet, that you're getting away with something. No, you are cheating yourself. If it's the way you want to eat and want to live, then it's the way to eat and live every day. With The Three Rules, a cheat day removes a critical part of the plan, All or None. Too often, a cheat day leads to repeated, more frequent breaking of The Rules.

Why don't you have a cheat day for your spouse? Why is an alcoholic not advised to have whiskey every other Thursday? Why is a gambling addict not supposed to play blackjack in Las Vegas on his birthday? Just as one whiskey leads to six and one hand of blackjack leads to hours of losses, one day of junk food leads to weight gain. All your efforts are wasted. The simple fact is that an alcoholic can't stop at one drink. If we could stop with one cheat day, we wouldn't have a weight problem.

What is the end you have in mind? Your goal should not be to complete a diet. Your goal should be to lose weight and keep it off. I do push-ups nearly every day to increase strength and endurance. My son watched me doing them and said, "You're cheating." I watched a video, and he was right. I wasn't doing full push-ups. My goal was not to do a certain number of push-ups but to get in better shape. I improved my form, having to cut my numbers in half, but I am better for it. Losing weight is the same. Is your goal to finish a diet plan, or is it to lose weight? No one is watching you and giving you a grade. If the end you have in mind is weight control, don't cheat yourself.

Saboteurs

Saboteurs are people who intentionally or unintentionally hinder your diet plan. It is unlikely that you have friends who consciously want you to fail, but you will run into those who make it more difficult for you. At home, they will bring doughnuts, bagels (treats in my family), and other junk food. In the office, they will bring treats or invite you to lunch at a pizza place. At a party or restaurant, they will keep asking you to try the dessert.

We've discussed how to handle gifts and similar temptations to stray from The Rules, but sometimes the saboteur is more aggressive. They may openly tell you that you're being too restrictive or that you have to "live a little." I used to say and still sometimes think, "I want to live a lot longer, so I eat this way." I don't recommend that. I suggest, "No, thanks." If they persist, say it again. If they keep pushing, say nothing or something like, "This is how I want to live. I feel it's the best for me."

That usually ends it. If not, then they may not be the friend you thought they were. Consider a more extended conversation or even distancing yourself from them. If they push you this hard, there could be more animosity than you think, and you're unlikely to have a good relationship in the future. Alternatively, if you believe their behavior is motivated by something within themselves, such as low self-esteem, perhaps you could help them work on it. If they're overweight, they may envy your strength in dealing with it, and you could ask them to join you in The Three Rules.

What To Do If (When) You Slip Up?

Rarely does anyone embark on a plan and never make a mistake. Most reformed alcoholics slip a few times. The same is true with The Three Rules. Over the years, I've slipped more than a few times. Whether you succeed after a lapse depends on what you do next. I learned from *The Willpower Instinct* that we should imagine failure so that we will have a plan in place. I do that myself and recommended it to patients. If you have a plan for what to do, you are less likely to feel bad about yourself after the slip-up, and feeling bad leads to eating unhealthy foods. Make a plan and state it plainly. "If I eat something against The Rules, I will…" My plan is always to start again the moment I finish. I don't wait until the following day. Then, it is too easy to extend the mistake for days on end. If I'm back on The Rules immediately, I feel good about myself for having made only one mistake. There is less risk of the snowball effect of guilt followed by more eating. Try your hardest to follow The Rules. If you don't intend to eat a treat but eat it anyway, follow your plan and return to The Rules.

Conclusion
and Final Thoughts

Today is the best day to start anything.

The Three Rules to Lose Weight and Keep It Off Forever will help you control your weight. But you will do the work. You will learn and become a better person for it. It takes hard work. You can do it. Do not start on this or any plan unless you are ready to commit to it, prepared to do the work it takes, and willing to follow through.

Experts discuss the importance of changing your lifestyle rather than starting a diet. To me, lifestyle is something superficial and visible to others. I prefer to think of The Three Rules as a way of living. Eat with intent. Choose to eat what is good for your life or to eat whatever you want, regardless of the consequences. But do it on purpose. If it's worth eating only healthy foods, it is worth eating that way every day, like brushing your teeth, showering, and not smoking. Over the years, I often heard patients tell me they don't smoke or drink, and when I asked them when they quit, they said, "Today." I used to laugh. But really, that is all there is to making a change. Quit eating junk food and bad carbs today. Eat with intent starting today. Tomorrow, do the same thing. Then you are done.

We should do everything important with intent, thinking about whether it is right for our lives. Whether you eat a cupcake on any given day seems too minor to think about in these terms, but that is how life is. It is made up of choices and decisions that we make right now. We are living right now, not in the future or the past.

Many things in our lives, most things in fact, are beyond our control. I will never have a full head of hair, play basketball well, remember everything I read, or be a concert pianist. I can only control my mind and how I act in a situation. I can control my temper when someone cuts me off in traffic. I can smile when I meet a stranger. I can work to become a better writer. I can abstain from alcohol. I can exercise regularly. And I can control what I eat today.

The Serenity Prayer has existed in various forms for generations. We pray or ask for the serenity to accept the things we cannot change, the courage to change the things we can, and the wisdom to know the difference. We should apply this message to every day of our lives, including our health and how we eat. It is straightforward as to losing weight and keeping it off. You have the wisdom to know that you can lose weight because all it takes is to give up bad carbs and junk food. It takes courage to change and give up these foods forever. I believe you have that courage. If you make the commitment, starting now, you will succeed. You will lose weight and change your life forever.

About The Author

Harold Oster recently retired from his medical practice in Plymouth, Minnesota. He went to medical school in Miami, Florida, did his residency in San Diego, and returned to Miami to study Infectious Diseases. Given his propensity to gain weight, he has become interested in obesity and weight management. You can visit his business website at haroldoster.com.

www.ingramcontent.com/pod-product-compliance
Lightning Source LLC
Chambersburg PA
CBHW071510140726
47997CB00005B/1924